Thyroid Wellness Blueprint

The Ultimate Guide to Understanding, Managing, and Thriving Despite the Challenges of Thyroid Disorders

Tamie Larson

Copyright © 2024 by Tamie Larson

About the Author

Tamie Larson, MD, stands at the forefront of thyroid health, bringing a wealth of expertise and insight into the management and treatment of thyroid disorders. With a distinguished medical degree and specialized training in endocrinology, Dr. Larson has dedicated her career to advancing the understanding and care of thyroid-related health issues.

Dr. Larson's journey into the world of thyroidology began during her residency, where she developed a profound interest in the complexities of thyroid disorders. Her passion for the field grew as she gained extensive hands-on experience, coupled with a relentless commitment to keeping pace with the latest medical breakthroughs. Today, she is celebrated as a leading authority in the realm of thyroid health, particularly noted for her work with autoimmune thyroid disorders.

Renowned for her empathetic and patient-centered approach, Dr. Larson extends her expertise beyond conventional medical treatments. She emphasizes the importance of holistic health practices, understanding the deep interconnection between thyroid function and overall well-being. Her approach to patient care is comprehensive, incorporating both advanced medical treatments and lifestyle modifications to achieve the best outcomes.

In addition to her clinical practice, Dr. Larson is an esteemed educator and public speaker. Her contributions to medical conferences and seminars have significantly enriched the discourse in thyroidology and autoimmune health. She is also a passionate advocate for patient education and empowerment, a commitment that shines through in her writing and public engagements.

"Thyroid Wellness Blueprint" is a culmination of Dr. Tamie Larson's years of expertise and dedication. This book is crafted to be a valuable resource for anyone seeking to navigate the challenges of thyroid disorders. Readers will find a treasure trove of knowledge and practical advice, making complex medical concepts accessible and manageable. Dr. Larson's work is more than a guide; it is a companion for those on their journey to achieving optimal thyroid health and wellness.

Table of Contents

Introduction

As a seasoned thyroidologist, my journey through the complex world of thyroid disorders has been both professionally enriching and personally humbling. I have had the privilege of working closely with many who have battled these conditions, and their resilience and strength have inspired me to pen "Thyroid Wellness Blueprint." This book is not just a culmination of medical knowledge and research; it is a testament to the human spirit's ability to persevere and triumph in the face of health challenges.

The significance of the thyroid gland in our overall health cannot be overstated. This small, butterfly-shaped gland nestled in our neck has profound effects that ripple throughout the body. It controls metabolism, influences heart rate, regulates temperature, and even impacts mood. When the thyroid malfunctions, it isn't merely a disruption of a singular system; it's a disturbance that can affect every aspect of one's life. Conditions such as hypothyroidism and hyperthyroidism can lead to a cascade of physical and emotional changes, ranging from extreme fatigue and weight fluctuations to anxiety and depression.

In writing "Thyroid Wellness Blueprint," I aim to demystify the complexities surrounding thyroid disorders. Throughout my practice, I have encountered countless myths and misconceptions about these conditions. There is a widespread belief that thyroid disorders are easy to diagnose and treat, or that they exclusively affect a certain demographic. This book seeks to dispel such myths, offering clarity and insight into the true nature of thyroid disorders. It's vital to understand that thyroid health is nuanced and that each individual's journey is unique.

This book is structured to provide a comprehensive guide through the labyrinth of thyroid health. It starts with the basics – explaining the function of the thyroid gland and its paramount role in our body's metabolism. We then delve deeper into the various thyroid disorders, exploring their causes, symptoms, and the latest advancements in their treatment. Recognizing the importance of holistic care, the book also covers lifestyle and dietary recommendations, delving into how daily habits can significantly impact thyroid health.

Each chapter is meticulously crafted to build upon the last, ensuring a seamless flow of information. Whether you are newly diagnosed with a thyroid condition, a long-term sufferer, a caregiver, or a healthcare professional, this book is designed to cater to a broad spectrum of readers. Its content is meant to enlighten, guide, and provide solace, offering both scientific knowledge and practical advice.

Furthermore, "Thyroid Wellness Blueprint" acknowledges the emotional and psychological toll of living with a thyroid disorder. It offers strategies for coping, advice on building a strong support network, and tips for maintaining mental and emotional wellness. The book emphasizes the importance of patient empowerment and self-advocacy, encouraging readers to take an active role in their health journey.

As you turn each page, I hope you find more than just facts and guidelines. My aspiration is for this book to be a source of comfort, a beacon of hope, and a tool for empowerment. I want readers to feel equipped to navigate the challenges of thyroid disorders, armed with knowledge and reassured by the shared experiences and insights from others who have walked this path.

In conclusion, "Thyroid Wellness Blueprint" is more than just a medical guide; it's a companion on your journey towards better health. It's a bridge between the medical community and those affected by thyroid disorders, fostering understanding, compassion, and most importantly, hope. As you embark on this journey with me, know that you are not alone. Together, we can navigate the complexities of thyroid health and strive toward a life of balance, wellness, and vitality.

Chapter One: Thyroid Basics

In this chapter, we embark on a foundational journey to understand the thyroid gland—a key player in our body's intricate system. Here, we'll explore the anatomy and function of the thyroid, revealing how this small gland has a colossal impact on our overall health. We'll delve into the production and regulation of thyroid hormones, vital agents that orchestrate a myriad of bodily functions.

Understanding these processes is crucial, as it leads us to identify and comprehend thyroid imbalances—conditions that affect countless individuals worldwide. Furthermore, we'll highlight the significance of maintaining thyroid health, not just for physical well-being but for our holistic health. This chapter lays the groundwork for understanding the complexities and importance of thyroid health, setting the stage for deeper insights in subsequent chapters.

Understanding Thyroid Anatomy and Function

The thyroid gland, an essential part of the human endocrine system, plays a pivotal role in regulating a wide range of metabolic processes that are crucial for maintaining overall health and well-being. This small, butterfly-shaped gland, strategically located in the lower front part of the neck, below the Adam's apple and encircling the trachea, is both a powerhouse and a master regulator. Comprising two lobes connected by a thin strip of tissue known as the isthmus, its placement at the base of the neck allows it to efficiently release hormones directly into the bloodstream.

Richly supplied with blood vessels, the thyroid gland is uniquely positioned to ensure the rapid transport of hormones to various body tissues. It's intricately intertwined with other vital structures in the neck, such as the parathyroid glands and recurrent laryngeal nerves, which highlights the complexity and delicacy of this area. The gland is encapsulated in a delicate connective tissue, further emphasizing the precision required in thyroid surgeries.

The thyroid's primary function is to produce, store, and release two key hormones: thyroxine (T4) and triiodothyronine (T3). These hormones are indispensable in regulating the body's metabolism, growth, and development. T4, the main hormone produced, accounts for about 90% of thyroid hormone production and functions as a prohormone. It has a lower activity level and needs to be converted into the more active T3 in various body tissues. This conversion process allows for a regulated release of the active hormone, facilitating the body's various metabolic needs.

T3, though produced in smaller quantities, is significantly more potent than T4. It acts rapidly and has pronounced effects on the body. The synthesis of these hormones is a sophisticated process involving iodine, an essential element absorbed from the diet. The thyroid cells are specially equipped to absorb, store, and use iodine for hormone synthesis, a unique feature that sets them apart from other cells in the body.

The influence of thyroid hormones extends across the body. They regulate the basal metabolic rate, affecting how the body uses energy. By stimulating various metabolic activities, these hormones play a vital role in processes like heat generation, oxygen consumption, and energy expenditure. In children and adolescents, thyroid hormones are crucial for normal growth and development, especially in terms of brain development and bone growth. Any imbalance in these hormones can lead to significant developmental delays.

Moreover, thyroid hormones have a substantial impact on the cardiovascular system. They enhance cardiac output by increasing the heart rate and the force of cardiac muscle contractions, thus influencing blood pressure and overall cardiac function. Beyond physical health, these hormones are integral to brain function, affecting aspects such as mood, cognition, and nerve function. Imbalances in thyroid hormone levels can lead to mood disorders and cognitive impairments, illustrating their significance in neurological health.

The thyroid hormones also regulate other body systems, including the digestive and reproductive systems, and influence muscle function. This broad range of influence underscores the importance of maintaining optimal thyroid health for overall physiological and psychological well-being. Understanding the anatomy and function of the thyroid gland is therefore crucial, as it forms the foundation for comprehending the myriad ways in which thyroid imbalances can manifest and affect the human body.

Thyroid Hormone Production and Regulation

The synthesis and regulation of thyroid hormones are vital processes for maintaining metabolic equilibrium and overall bodily function. These complex processes hinge on the functionality of the thyroid gland, an organ characterized by its butterfly shape located at the front of the neck, just below the Adam's apple. Understanding the detailed steps of hormone synthesis and the regulatory mechanisms that control this process is fundamental for both the comprehension and management of thyroid-related disorders.

The journey of thyroid hormone synthesis begins with iodide, a key ingredient that the body obtains from dietary sources. Once ingested, iodide enters the bloodstream and is transported to the thyroid gland. Here, it is actively taken up by follicular cells of the thyroid via a protein known as the sodium-iodide symporter. This iodide is then transported into the colloid of the follicles, where it undergoes oxidation by the enzyme thyroid peroxidase (TPO), converting it into its reactive form, iodine. The iodine is then ready to be attached to the amino acid tyrosine, which is embedded in a large protein called thyroglobulin, a process known as organification.

Thyroglobulin, synthesized by the follicular cells and secreted into the colloid, serves as a scaffold for thyroid hormone synthesis. Iodine attaches to tyrosine residues on thyroglobulin to form monoiodotyrosine (MIT) and diiodotyrosine (DIT). The coupling of these iodotyrosines is the next critical step: two DIT molecules join to form Thyroxine (T4), while one DIT and one MIT molecule combine to form Triiodothyronine (T3). These hormones remain part of the thyroglobulin molecule until they are released into the bloodstream.

When the body requires thyroid hormones, thyroglobulin is endocytosed back into the follicular cells and merged with lysosomes. Lysosomal enzymes cleave the T4 and T3 from the thyroglobulin, releasing them into the bloodstream. It's noteworthy that while the thyroid gland primarily produces T4, it's the conversion of T4 into the more active T3 in peripheral tissues, a process facilitated by deiodinase enzymes, that is predominantly responsible for the active thyroid hormone effects in the body.

The regulation of this synthesis process is meticulously controlled by the hypothalamic-pituitary-thyroid axis. This axis involves a feedback loop with the hypothalamus and the pituitary gland, two master regulators located in the brain. The hypothalamus monitors thyroid hormone levels and responds by secreting Thyrotropin-releasing hormone (TRH) when it detects a need for more thyroid hormones. TRH then stimulates the pituitary gland to release Thyroid-stimulating hormone (TSH), which directly acts on the thyroid gland.

TSH is the key hormone in regulating thyroid function, stimulating every step of thyroid hormone synthesis, including iodide uptake, iodination of tyrosine, and the release of T4 and T3 from thyroglobulin. The levels of TSH released by the pituitary gland are in turn regulated by the levels of circulating thyroid hormones in a classic negative feedback loop. High levels of circulating T4 and T3 inhibit the release of TRH and TSH, decreasing thyroid hormone production. Conversely, low levels of circulating thyroid hormones stimulate the production of TRH and TSH, thus increasing thyroid hormone production.

This feedback loop ensures a balance of thyroid hormones in the body, adapting to the body's needs and protecting against both under and overproduction of hormones. Disruptions in this finely tuned regulatory mechanism can lead to various forms of thyroid dysfunction, including hypothyroidism, where there is too little thyroid hormone, or hyperthyroidism, with too much hormone. Each condition presents its spectrum of symptoms and requires specific management strategies.

In summary, the production and regulation of thyroid hormones are intricate processes that are critical for maintaining a wide range of bodily functions. The thyroid gland, through its synthesis of T4 and T3, regulates metabolism, growth, development, and many other processes. The hypothalamic-pituitary-thyroid axis ensures the proper regulation of these hormones, maintaining homeostasis. Understanding these processes provides invaluable insights into the functioning of the human body and the importance of thyroid health in overall well-being. This knowledge forms the basis for diagnosing, managing, and treating various thyroid disorders, highlighting the significance of the thyroid gland in human health.

Identifying Thyroid Imbalances

Identifying thyroid imbalances is a critical aspect of managing thyroid health, requiring an awareness of the diverse and sometimes subtle symptoms associated with hypo- and hyperthyroidism. These conditions, stemming from underactivity or overactivity of the thyroid gland, can significantly affect various bodily functions.

Symptoms of Hypothyroidism

Hypothyroidism is characterized by a deficiency in thyroid hormone production, leading to a general slowing down of the body's metabolic processes. Symptoms often develop slowly and can be mistaken for the normal aging process. They include:

Persistent Fatigue and Lethargy: One of the most common symptoms, characterized by an overall lack of energy and a constant feeling of tiredness.

Unexplained Weight Gain: Weight gain may occur, often despite maintaining a typical diet and exercise routine.

Increased Sensitivity to Cold: Individuals may find themselves intolerant to colder temperatures, needing extra layers or heating.

Dry and Rough Skin, Brittle Hair: The skin may become unusually dry and rough, and hair can turn brittle, coarse, and subject to more hair loss.

Constipation: Slowed digestive processes can lead to chronic constipation.

Depressive Mood States: Mood disturbances, particularly depression, are commonly associated with hypothyroidism.

Cognitive Difficulties: Experiencing problems with memory, focus, and concentration.

Menstrual Changes and Fertility Issues: Women might face irregular, heavy menstrual periods and problems with fertility.

Bradycardia (Slowed Heart Rate): A noticeable decrease in heart rate can occur.

Musculoskeletal Complaints: Joint and muscle pain, stiffness, and tenderness, along with general weakness, can be prominent.

Elevated Blood Cholesterol Levels: Hypothyroidism can lead to high cholesterol levels, increasing the risk for heart disease.

Puffy Face and Hoarseness: Swelling of the face and a hoarse voice are less common but notable symptoms.

Impaired Hearing: Some individuals may experience a degree of hearing loss.

Symptoms of Hyperthyroidism

Hyperthyroidism results from an overproduction of thyroid hormones, leading to an acceleration of the body's metabolic rate. Symptoms are often more abrupt and can include:

Sudden Weight Loss: Rapid weight loss, despite normal or increased appetite.

Hyperthermia (Heat Intolerance): Difficulty tolerating warm temperatures and excessive sweating.

Palpitations and Tachycardia: Rapid heartbeat, sometimes accompanied by irregular heart rhythms or palpitations.

Nervousness, Anxiety, and Irritability: Psychological effects including mood swings, nervousness, and heightened anxiety.

Tremors: Fine shaking, particularly noticeable in the hands.

Altered Menstrual Patterns in Women: Lighter, less frequent menstruation.

Increased Bowel Movements: Diarrhea or increased frequency in bowel movements.

Goiter (Thyroid Enlargement): Visible swelling in the neck due to thyroid enlargement.

Muscle Weakness and Fatigue: Despite increased energy levels, individuals may experience overall fatigue and weakness, particularly in the upper arms and thighs.

Sleep Disturbances: Difficulty in falling or staying asleep.

Skin Changes: Skin may become thin and fragile.

Eye Problems: Especially in Graves' disease, symptoms like bulging eyes, redness, and irritation can occur.

Other Indicators of Thyroid Dysfunction

Apart from the classic symptoms, other signs can indicate thyroid dysfunction:

Hoarseness and Neck Discomfort: Enlargement of the thyroid can cause a change in voice and a feeling of tightness in the throat.

High Cholesterol Levels: Particularly in hypothyroidism, unexpectedly high cholesterol levels can be a red flag.

Breathing and Swallowing Difficulties: In cases of significant goiter, there can be difficulty in breathing or swallowing.

Heart Problems: Both hypo- and hyperthyroidism can lead to various heart-related issues, including atrial fibrillation, cardiomyopathy, and others.

Mental Health Issues: Beyond depression in hypothyroidism, both conditions can lead to anxiety, mood swings, and other psychiatric symptoms.

Eye Abnormalities: Apart from bulging eyes in Graves' disease, there can be puffiness, dry eyes, and vision problems.

Identifying these symptoms is crucial for timely and accurate diagnosis of thyroid disorders. Often, a combination of clinical assessment and blood tests measuring thyroid hormone (T3 and T4) and thyroid-stimulating hormone (TSH) levels are used to confirm the diagnosis. Given the broad spectrum of symptoms, thyroid imbalances can sometimes be misdiagnosed or overlooked, underscoring the importance of thorough and regular medical evaluations for those experiencing such signs. Early detection and management are key to preventing complications and maintaining optimal health.

Importance of Thyroid Health

The thyroid gland, a small but vital part of the endocrine system, plays a crucial role in regulating numerous bodily functions. Its impact on the body is extensive, influencing various systems and holding significant implications for long-term health.

Thyroid hormones, particularly thyroxine (T4) and triiodothyronine (T3) are essential in regulating the body's metabolic rate. These hormones have a profound influence on the cardiovascular system. They regulate heart rate, blood pressure, and cholesterol levels. In hypothyroidism, the reduced production of these hormones can lead to bradycardia (a slower heart rate), increased arterial stiffness, and elevated cholesterol levels. These changes heighten the risk of developing heart disease and atherosclerosis. Hyperthyroidism, on the other hand, can cause tachycardia (an increased heart rate), palpitations, and arrhythmias, which may escalate to heart failure if left untreated.

The influence of thyroid hormones extends to the digestive system as well. In hypothyroidism, a reduction in hormone levels can slow down gastrointestinal motility, leading to constipation and bloating. Hyperthyroidism can have the opposite effect, increasing the speed of digestion and leading to more frequent bowel movements or even diarrhea.

Reproductive health is also closely tied to thyroid function. In women, thyroid imbalances can lead to menstrual irregularities, changes in menstrual flow, and difficulties in conception. During pregnancy, uncontrolled thyroid conditions can lead to higher risks of miscarriage, preterm labor, and preeclampsia. For men, thyroid dysfunction can influence testosterone levels, potentially leading to reduced libido and issues with fertility.

The musculoskeletal system is significantly impacted by thyroid hormones. In children and adolescents, hypothyroidism can lead to delayed bone growth and development. In adults, prolonged periods of hypo- or hyperthyroidism can contribute to osteoporosis, increasing the risk of fractures and other bone-related issues due to altered bone remodeling processes.

One of the most critical roles of thyroid hormones is in the development and function of the nervous system. Hypothyroidism can lead to symptoms such as depression, mental fog, memory problems, and a general slowing of cognitive functions. Conversely, hyperthyroidism can result in symptoms like anxiety, irritability, and nervousness. In severe cases, untreated hypothyroidism can result in a life-threatening condition called myxedema coma, characterized by extreme drowsiness, hypothermia, and unconsciousness. Similarly, untreated hyperthyroidism can lead to a thyrotoxic crisis (thyroid storm), a dangerous condition marked by fever, delirium, and severe tachycardia.

The long-term health implications of thyroid dysfunction are substantial. Chronic cardiovascular issues such as hypertension, heart disease, and the risk of heart attacks and strokes are associated with long-standing hypothyroidism. Untreated hyperthyroidism can lead to persistent high blood pressure, arrhythmias, and a heightened risk of heart failure. Both hypo- and hyperthyroidism can lead to serious bone health issues, including an increased risk of osteoporosis and fractures, especially in postmenopausal women and the elderly.

Thyroid disorders can also have profound effects on mental health. Persistent depressive states and cognitive decline are common in hypothyroidism, while anxiety disorders and insomnia are often associated with hyperthyroidism. During pregnancy, improperly managed thyroid disorders can lead to complications that affect both the mother and the fetus, including developmental issues, miscarriage, and preterm birth.

Moreover, the overall quality of life can be severely impacted by chronic thyroid dysfunction. Symptoms such as fatigue, mood disturbances, and impaired physical and cognitive abilities can affect daily activities, work productivity, and personal relationships. The psychological burden of living with a chronic condition, along with the physical symptoms, can lead to decreased life satisfaction and mental health issues.

Therefore, recognizing the importance of thyroid health is crucial. Regular monitoring of thyroid function, especially in individuals with symptoms or a family history of thyroid disorders, is key to early detection and effective management. Appropriate treatment and lifestyle modifications can significantly mitigate the risk of long-term complications, ensuring a better quality of life and maintaining overall health and well-being. This comprehensive approach to thyroid health is essential for preventing severe health complications and promoting a healthier, more fulfilling life.

Chapter Two: Hypothyroidism - The Underactive Thyroid

In this chapter, we delve into the often-misunderstood world of hypothyroidism, a condition where the thyroid gland fails to produce sufficient hormones. This in-depth exploration begins with a comprehensive look at hypothyroidism, unraveling its symptoms and the way it silently affects various aspects of health. We then examine the causes and risk factors, revealing why some individuals are more susceptible to this condition.

The chapter progresses to the critical aspects of diagnosing hypothyroidism, discussing the tests and indicators that aid in its detection. Finally, we focus on the treatment strategies, encompassing both medical interventions and lifestyle adjustments, to effectively manage and mitigate the impacts of this condition. This chapter aims to provide clarity and guidance for those navigating the complexities of an underactive thyroid.

Understanding Hypothyroidism

Hypothyroidism, also known as an underactive thyroid, is a condition characterized by the insufficient production of thyroid hormones by the thyroid gland. These hormones, thyroxine (T4) and triiodothyronine (T3) are crucial regulators of the body's metabolism. When the thyroid gland does not produce adequate levels of these hormones, it leads to a slowdown in various bodily functions and metabolic processes.

Definition of Hypothyroidism

The thyroid gland, located at the base of the neck, plays a pivotal role in regulating numerous physiological processes. Thyroid hormones influence growth, development, and cellular repair, as well as metabolic functions like energy expenditure, heat production, and heart rate regulation. In hypothyroidism, the deficiency in T3 and T4 results in a widespread reduction in metabolic activities, causing symptoms such as persistent fatigue, unexplained weight gain, intolerance to cold temperatures, and mood disturbances including depression.

The impact of hypothyroidism extends to multiple organ systems. For instance, the reduced metabolic rate can cause bradycardia (slowed heart rate) and elevated cholesterol levels, increasing the risk for atherosclerosis and other heart diseases. The gastrointestinal system may slow down, leading to constipation. Neurologically, individuals may experience memory issues, slowed thinking, and depressive symptoms. Women often face menstrual irregularities and potential fertility issues, while men might experience reduced libido.

The onset of hypothyroidism symptoms is typically gradual, and they can be subtle in the initial stages, sometimes making early diagnosis challenging. Over time, these symptoms become more pronounced and may significantly impact the quality of life.

Types of Hypothyroidism

Hypothyroidism can be categorized into several types, each with distinct causes and characteristics:

Primary Hypothyroidism: This is the most common form where the dysfunction lies in the thyroid gland itself. It can result from autoimmune conditions like Hashimoto's thyroiditis, where the immune system attacks the thyroid, leading to inflammation and reduced hormone production. Other causes include iodine deficiency, certain medications, radiation therapy, and thyroid surgery.

Secondary Hypothyroidism: In this less common form, the problem arises from the pituitary gland, which fails to produce sufficient thyroid-stimulating hormone (TSH) necessary for thyroid hormone production. It can result from pituitary tumors, head trauma, or pituitary gland diseases.

Tertiary Hypothyroidism: This rare type is due to a lack of thyrotropin-releasing hormone (TRH) from the hypothalamus, which is necessary for stimulating TSH production in the pituitary gland. Causes can include hypothalamic disease, injury, or tumors.

Congenital Hypothyroidism: Present from birth, this occurs when the thyroid gland is absent, ectopic (not located in the normal position), or underdeveloped. Early detection and treatment are crucial to prevent intellectual disability and growth failure.

Subclinical Hypothyroidism: This mild or early form is characterized by normal levels of T3 and T4 but elevated TSH levels. Some people may exhibit negligible symptoms or none at all.

Iatrogenic Hypothyroidism: This type results from medical treatments that affect thyroid function, such as thyroidectomy (surgical removal of the thyroid gland) or radioactive iodine treatment for hyperthyroidism.

Each type of hypothyroidism has its unique causal factors and may necessitate different diagnostic and therapeutic approaches. Proper understanding and classification of the specific type of hypothyroidism are essential for effective treatment and management. This includes tailored hormone replacement therapy and addressing the underlying cause of the thyroid dysfunction.

Causes and Risk Factors

Hypothyroidism, characterized by reduced thyroid hormone production, is influenced by a complex interplay of factors, including autoimmune processes, environmental influences, genetic predisposition, and various health conditions. Understanding these factors in detail is crucial for the effective identification, treatment, and management of this condition.

Autoimmune Causes: Hashimoto's Thyroiditis

The predominant cause of hypothyroidism, especially in iodine-sufficient regions, is Hashimoto's thyroiditis. This is an autoimmune disorder where the immune system erroneously targets and gradually destroys the thyroid gland.

Hashimoto's Thyroiditis: The immune response in this condition leads to the production of antibodies against thyroid tissue. The resulting inflammation damages the thyroid cells, diminishing their ability to produce hormones. Initially, this may cause the thyroid gland to enlarge (forming a goiter), but over time, the gland often becomes shrunken and fibrotic, leading to a chronic deficiency in thyroid hormone production.

Environmental and Genetic Factors

Numerous environmental and genetic factors also significantly contribute to the risk and development of hypothyroidism:

Iodine Intake: Iodine is essential for thyroid hormone synthesis. Both deficiency and excess can lead to hypothyroidism. Iodine deficiency is a common cause in areas with low iodine levels in the diet, leading to reduced hormone production. Excessive iodine can also disrupt thyroid function, though this is less frequent.

Radiation Exposure: Exposure to radiation, especially in the neck or head region, can harm the thyroid gland. This includes radiation treatments for cancers and exposure to environmental radiation (like nuclear accidents). The damage can impair the gland's ability to produce hormones.

Medication Effects: Certain drugs are known to affect thyroid function. Lithium, used in bipolar disorder, and amiodarone, used for heart rhythm problems, can induce hypothyroidism. Other drugs, such as interferon-alpha, interleukin-2, and some types of chemotherapy, may also have similar effects.

Thyroid Surgery and Treatments: Hypothyroidism can be a direct consequence of surgical removal of the thyroid gland or parts of it. Likewise, radioactive iodine treatment, typically used for hyperthyroidism, often leads to a reduction in thyroid function.

Genetic Factors: There's a hereditary component to hypothyroidism. The risk increases in individuals with a family history of thyroid disease. Specific gene mutations, some of which have been identified, can predispose individuals to thyroid dysfunction.

Pregnancy: Some women develop hypothyroidism during or after pregnancy due to the complex hormonal and immunological changes that occur. This condition is often temporary but can sometimes evolve into permanent hypothyroidism.

Associated Autoimmune Conditions: The presence of other autoimmune diseases such as Type 1 diabetes, rheumatoid arthritis, lupus, or celiac disease can increase the likelihood of developing autoimmune thyroid diseases, including Hashimoto's thyroiditis.

Age and Gender: Hypothyroidism is more prevalent among older adults, particularly in women. Women, especially those over the age of 60, are at a higher risk compared to men.

Inflammatory Thyroiditis: Inflammation of the thyroid gland, which can occur due to viral infections (subacute thyroiditis) or after pregnancy (postpartum thyroiditis), can impair thyroid function temporarily or permanently.

Environmental Toxins: Certain environmental chemicals and toxins, such as perchlorate, polychlorinated biphenyls (PCBs), and heavy metals, can interfere with thyroid hormone production and regulation.

Dietary Factors: Some dietary components can impact thyroid function. High consumption of soy products and cruciferous vegetables (like broccoli and cauliflower) can affect thyroid hormone synthesis, especially in those with existing iodine deficiency.

Smoking: Smoking tobacco has been associated with an increased risk of thyroid disease. Certain compounds in tobacco smoke can interfere with thyroid function and may exacerbate autoimmune thyroid diseases.

By recognizing these diverse causes and risk factors, healthcare professionals can better identify individuals at risk for hypothyroidism and provide more targeted screening and intervention strategies. This comprehensive understanding is vital for preventing the progression of the condition and minimizing its impact on health and quality of life.

Diagnosing Hypothyroidism

Diagnosing hypothyroidism, a condition where the thyroid gland is underactive and produces insufficient thyroid hormones, involves a meticulous approach combining clinical evaluation and a series of diagnostic tests. This process aims to accurately assess thyroid function and distinguish hypothyroidism from other conditions that might present with similar symptoms.

Blood Tests and Interpretation

The diagnosis of hypothyroidism primarily revolves around blood tests that measure various aspects of thyroid function:

TSH Test (Thyroid-Stimulating Hormone): This test is typically the first step in thyroid evaluation. TSH is produced by the pituitary gland and stimulates the thyroid to produce thyroxine (T4) and triiodothyronine (T3). In primary hypothyroidism, the thyroid gland's decreased hormone production leads to compensatory elevated TSH levels. A high TSH level, especially when coupled with low thyroid hormone levels, is a primary indicator of hypothyroidism.

Free T4 (Thyroxine) Test: Free T4 testing measures the unbound, active form of T4 in the blood. The primary hormone that the thyroid gland produces is T4. Low levels of free T4 are a hallmark of hypothyroidism and help confirm the diagnosis suggested by elevated TSH levels.

Free T3 Test: Though T3 testing is less commonly used in initial hypothyroidism screening, it can be valuable in certain clinical scenarios. T3 is the active form of thyroid hormone, and its levels can provide additional insight, especially in complex cases.

Thyroid Antibody Tests: In autoimmune thyroiditis (Hashimoto's thyroiditis), the body produces antibodies against thyroid tissue, leading to chronic inflammation and impaired hormone production. Testing for thyroid peroxidase antibodies (TPOAb) and thyroglobulin antibodies (TgAb) can confirm an autoimmune process. The presence of these antibodies is indicative of Hashimoto's thyroiditis, a common cause of hypothyroidism.

Additional Diagnostic Tools and Considerations

Apart from blood tests, other tools and considerations are employed to obtain a comprehensive picture of thyroid health:

Ultrasound of the Thyroid: An ultrasound provides detailed imaging of the thyroid gland, revealing structural characteristics like volume, presence of nodules, or signs of inflammation. It's particularly useful for detecting goiters or thyroid growths, common in various thyroid disorders, including hypothyroidism.

Radioiodine Uptake Test: This nuclear medicine test evaluates how well the thyroid gland absorbs iodine from the bloodstream. It can provide insights into thyroid function by measuring the gland's ability to take up iodine, which is critical for hormone production. Although more typically used in hyperthyroidism diagnosis, it can occasionally aid in understanding certain hypothyroidism cases.

Thyroid Scan: Involving a radioactive tracer, a thyroid scan can visualize the gland's activity, showing areas of low or high activity. It's particularly useful when other tests provide ambiguous results.

Pituitary and Hypothalamic Function Tests: If secondary or tertiary hypothyroidism (issues stemming from the pituitary or hypothalamus) is suspected, tests to evaluate these areas of the brain may be conducted. This can include measuring other pituitary hormones or employing imaging studies like MRI to look for pituitary or hypothalamic tumors.

Basal Body Temperature Assessment: Historically, basal body temperature was used as a crude measure of metabolic rate, indirectly indicating thyroid function. Though it's not a reliable diagnostic tool for hypothyroidism, it might provide adjunctive information in some cases.

Lipid Profile: Since hypothyroidism can affect cholesterol metabolism, leading to elevated cholesterol levels, a lipid profile might indirectly suggest thyroid dysfunction. However, this is not a diagnostic test for hypothyroidism but can indicate a need for thyroid function evaluation.

Complete Blood Count (CBC): A CBC can help identify anemia or other hematological abnormalities that may accompany hypothyroidism.

Other Imaging Tests: In rare cases, where pituitary or hypothalamic disorders are suspected as the cause of hypothyroidism, CT scans or MRIs may be used for detailed brain imaging.

Diagnosing hypothyroidism requires careful interpretation of these tests in conjunction with the patient's clinical symptoms and history.

Given the varied and often subtle nature of hypothyroidism symptoms, a thorough diagnostic approach is essential. Regular monitoring and reassessment are important, especially for individuals at risk or those showing subclinical or mild forms of thyroid dysfunction. Early and accurate diagnosis is key to managing hypothyroidism effectively, preventing complications, and ensuring optimal patient outcomes.

Treatment Strategies

Treating hypothyroidism, a condition characterized by an underactive thyroid gland producing insufficient amounts of essential hormones, necessitates a well-rounded approach that primarily involves hormone replacement therapy, complemented by lifestyle and dietary modifications. This comprehensive treatment strategy is designed to replenish the deficient hormone levels and address the various symptoms and complications associated with hypothyroidism.

The main treatment for hypothyroidism is hormone replacement therapy, typically with levothyroxine, a synthetic form of the thyroid hormone thyroxine (T4). This medication is integral in restoring the body's hormonal balance and normalizing metabolic functions disrupted by the hormone deficiency. Determining the correct dosage of levothyroxine is a delicate process, taking into account individual factors such as the patient's age, weight, the severity of the condition, and other existing health issues, particularly cardiac conditions.

For example, an older patient or someone with a history of heart disease may require a lower starting dose to minimize the strain on the heart. Regular blood tests to monitor levels of thyroid-stimulating hormone (TSH) and free T4 are essential in ensuring the effectiveness of the treatment and making necessary dosage adjustments. For most patients, levothyroxine therapy is a lifelong commitment, with the requirement for ongoing monitoring and dose adjustments, particularly in response to changes such as weight fluctuation, aging, pregnancy, or menopause.

In certain cases where patients do not experience adequate symptom relief from levothyroxine, alternative treatments may be considered. These can include liothyronine, a synthetic version of triiodothyronine (T3), or natural desiccated thyroid (NDT) extracts, which contain a combination of T3 and T4. These alternatives are generally used as second-line treatments under careful medical supervision, as they require close monitoring due to their potential to cause adverse effects.

In addition to pharmacotherapy, lifestyle and dietary modifications play a significant role in managing hypothyroidism. Engaging in regular physical activity is crucial for managing common symptoms like weight gain and fatigue and is beneficial for cardiovascular health. A balanced, nutrient-rich diet supports overall health and thyroid function. Adequate iodine intake is crucial, as it is necessary for thyroid hormone production, and can be achieved through a diet including seafood, dairy products, and iodized salt.

However, it is important to balance iodine intake as both deficiency and excess can affect thyroid function. Selenium and zinc, found in foods like Brazil nuts, seafood, meats, and legumes, are also important for thyroid health. Additionally, while certain foods known as goitrogens, like cruciferous vegetables, can interfere with thyroid function, their impact is minimal when cooked and consumed in moderation.

Managing stress through techniques like yoga, meditation, and mindfulness is important as stress can exacerbate thyroid disorders. It is also critical to ensure proper absorption of thyroid medication; levothyroxine should be taken on an empty stomach, and certain foods, supplements, and other medications that can interfere with its absorption should be avoided at the time of taking the medication.

Regular medical check-ups and thyroid function tests are key to ensuring the effectiveness of the treatment and making necessary adjustments. Additionally, quitting smoking is beneficial as smoking can negatively impact thyroid function and overall health. Due to the metabolic slowing associated with hypothyroidism, weight management through a balanced diet and regular exercise is important.

Overall, the effective management of hypothyroidism requires a combination of hormone replacement therapy and lifestyle and dietary adjustments. This approach not only helps normalize hormone levels but also enhances the overall quality of life for those affected by the condition. Regular consultations with healthcare providers are essential for monitoring the effectiveness of the treatment plan, making necessary adjustments, and preventing potential complications associated with hypothyroidism.

Chapter Three: Hyperthyroidism - The Overactive Thyroid

This chapter explores the complexities of hyperthyroidism, a condition characterized by excessive thyroid hormone production. We begin by delving into the fundamental aspects of understanding hyperthyroidism, shedding light on how this overactivity impacts the body. The chapter then navigates through the various causes and risk factors associated with hyperthyroidism, from autoimmune disorders to lifestyle influences.

We also discuss the diagnostic procedures employed to accurately identify this condition, including blood tests and imaging techniques. Finally, the focus shifts to the management of hyperthyroidism, outlining both medical treatments and lifestyle adjustments essential for controlling and alleviating the symptoms of this thyroid disorder.

Understanding Hyperthyroidism

Hyperthyroidism is a medical condition characterized by excessive production of thyroid hormones, thyroxine (T4) and triiodothyronine (T3), by the thyroid gland. This gland, located in the front of the neck, plays a pivotal role in regulating the body's metabolism. When it becomes overactive, it leads to an increased metabolic rate, affecting various physiological processes and leading to a range of symptoms.

The elevated levels of thyroid hormones in hyperthyroidism lead to an acceleration of metabolic processes. Individuals with hyperthyroidism typically experience a rapid heartbeat or palpitations, weight loss despite an increased appetite, and heightened nervousness or anxiety. Physical manifestations can include hand tremors, excessive sweating, heat intolerance, and more frequent bowel movements. Women may notice changes in their menstrual patterns, and other general symptoms include muscle weakness, difficulty sleeping, and changes in hair and skin texture.

From a psychological standpoint, hyperthyroidism can cause increased irritability, mood swings, and anxiety, and can negatively impact cognitive functions such as concentration and memory. It's also linked to exacerbation of cardiovascular issues, such as arrhythmias, and an increased risk of developing osteoporosis, especially in postmenopausal women.

Forms of Hyperthyroidism

There are several forms of hyperthyroidism, each with its own set of causes and characteristics:

Graves' Disease: This autoimmune disorder is the most common cause of hyperthyroidism. The body's immune system erroneously attacks the thyroid gland, leading it to produce excess hormones. Graves' disease is often associated with a goiter and can cause a distinctive eye condition known as Graves' ophthalmopathy or thyroid eye disease, where inflammation and other immune responses affect the eye muscles and tissue around the eyes, leading to symptoms like bulging eyes, discomfort, and potential vision problems.

Toxic Adenoma and Toxic Multinodular Goiter: These conditions result from one or more autonomously functioning nodules within the thyroid. These nodules produce thyroid hormones independently of the rest of the gland, leading to hyperthyroidism. While the nodules are typically benign, they can significantly affect the thyroid's hormone production.

Thyroiditis: This is an inflammation of the thyroid gland that can lead to excessive release of thyroid hormones, resulting in transient hyperthyroidism. Different types of thyroiditis exist, including postpartum thyroiditis, which occurs after giving birth, and subacute thyroiditis, which may follow a viral infection.

Excessive Iodine Intake: Iodine is a critical component used by the thyroid gland to produce hormones. An excess, which might come from certain medications, supplements, or dietary sources, can lead to hyperthyroidism, especially in individuals with pre-existing thyroid issues.

Overmedication with Thyroid Hormones: Patients treated for hypothyroidism with synthetic thyroid hormones might inadvertently receive too high a dose or might misuse the medication, leading to hyperthyroidism.

TSH-Secreting Pituitary Tumors: Although rare, some individuals might develop a tumor in the pituitary gland that secretes thyroid-stimulating hormone (TSH) independently, leading to excessive stimulation of the thyroid and hyperthyroidism.

Excessive Use of Thyroid Hormone Supplements: The misuse of thyroid hormone supplements, often for purposes like weight loss or enhancing athletic performance, can lead to hyperthyroidism.

Diagnosing and managing hyperthyroidism involves a comprehensive understanding of these various forms and their specific implications. Early detection is crucial for preventing the progression to more severe states such as thyroid storm, a life-threatening exacerbation of hyperthyroid symptoms. This condition is marked by a significant increase in heart rate, fever, and altered mental state, among other symptoms, and requires immediate medical intervention.

Causes and Risk Factors

Hyperthyroidism, marked by an overactive thyroid gland producing excess thyroid hormones, is influenced by a complex interplay of genetic, environmental, and lifestyle factors. A thorough understanding of these risk factors and triggers is essential for identifying individuals at higher risk, guiding preventive strategies, and ensuring effective management of the condition.

Genetic and autoimmune predispositions play a significant role in the development of hyperthyroidism. Individuals with a family history of thyroid disorders, particularly autoimmune thyroid diseases like Graves' disease, are at increased risk. This genetic susceptibility is often linked to specific genes involved in immune system functioning. Additionally, the presence of other autoimmune diseases, such as Type 1 diabetes, rheumatoid arthritis, or celiac disease, heightens the likelihood of developing autoimmune-related hyperthyroidism due to the common tendency of the immune system to malfunction in these conditions.

Gender and age are also key influencers in the risk of developing hyperthyroidism. The condition is notably more prevalent in women, likely due to hormonal influences on the immune system, making them more susceptible to autoimmune disorders. Hyperthyroidism most commonly affects individuals in their 20s to 40s, but it can occur at any age. In older adults, the symptoms of hyperthyroidism might be less obvious, potentially leading to underdiagnosis.

Lifestyle factors, particularly smoking, significantly increase the risk of hyperthyroidism. Smoking has been strongly associated with an increased risk of Graves' disease and can exacerbate the severity of associated eye problems, known as Graves' ophthalmopathy. The impact of emotional and physical stress as triggers for hyperthyroidism cannot be understated. Stress can disrupt immune function and hormonal balance, potentially triggering autoimmune reactions against the thyroid gland or exacerbating existing thyroid dysfunction.

Diet and nutrition, especially iodine intake, are crucial in thyroid health. The thyroid gland utilizes iodine to produce hormones, and excessive iodine consumption can precipitate hyperthyroidism, especially in individuals with pre-existing thyroid abnormalities. High dietary sources of iodine include certain seafood, seaweed, and iodine-containing supplements and medications.

Environmental factors, particularly radiation exposure, play a significant role in thyroid health. Exposure to radiation, especially during childhood or directed at the head and neck area, increases the risk of developing thyroid diseases, including hyperthyroidism. This risk is also evident in individuals exposed to environmental radiation, such as that from nuclear accidents.

Medications, such as amiodarone and interferon-alpha, are known to induce hyperthyroidism. Amiodarone, used for heart rhythm issues, is rich in iodine and can trigger thyroid dysfunction. Interferon-alpha, used in treating certain cancers and hepatitis C, can stimulate autoimmune responses against the thyroid gland.

Hormonal changes, particularly during pregnancy, the postpartum period, and menopause, can trigger or exacerbate thyroid issues. Pregnancy and the postpartum period involve significant hormonal shifts that can impact thyroid function. Some women may develop postpartum thyroiditis, which typically starts with a hyperthyroid phase. Menopausal hormonal changes can also influence thyroid function, though the link is less direct.

A history of thyroid surgery or radiotherapy to the neck region can alter thyroid function and potentially lead to hyperthyroidism. Additionally, overmedication with thyroid hormone replacements in patients with hypothyroidism can inadvertently result in hyperthyroidism.

Understanding these risk factors and triggers for hyperthyroidism is crucial. Individuals with these risk factors should be vigilant for symptoms and undergo regular medical screenings, including thyroid function tests. Lifestyle modifications, such as quitting smoking and managing stress, are beneficial in reducing the risk of developing hyperthyroidism. Early diagnosis and treatment are key to preventing the progression to more severe complications and improving overall health outcomes for those affected by hyperthyroidism.

Diagnosis of Hyperthyroidism

Diagnosing hyperthyroidism, a condition marked by excessive production of thyroid hormones by the thyroid gland necessitates a comprehensive and multifaceted approach. Physicians combine a series of blood tests, imaging techniques, and clinical evaluations to accurately diagnose the condition, understand its etiology, and determine the most effective treatment plan.

Blood Tests

Thyroid-Stimulating Hormone (TSH) Test: TSH is secreted by the pituitary gland and regulates the thyroid gland's production of hormones. In hyperthyroidism, the excess thyroid hormone typically suppresses TSH secretion, leading to undetectably low or significantly reduced TSH levels. This test is often the first line of investigation in suspected thyroid disorders due to its high sensitivity.

Free Thyroxine (Free T4) and Free Triiodothyronine (Free T3) Tests: These tests measure the levels of active thyroid hormones circulating in the blood. In hyperthyroidism, levels of Free T4 and/or Free T3 are typically elevated. These measurements are crucial for confirming the diagnosis and assessing the severity of the hyperthyroid state.

Thyroid Antibody Tests: Several antibodies can be involved in thyroid disorders. In Graves' disease, Thyroid Stimulating Immunoglobulin (TSI) or TSH Receptor Antibody (TRAb) are typically elevated. Thyroid Peroxidase Antibodies (TPOAb) can also be elevated in autoimmune thyroid conditions. These tests help determine the autoimmune nature of hyperthyroidism.

Imaging and Other Diagnostic Methods

Radioactive Iodine Uptake (RAIU) Test: This test measures how much radioactive iodine is absorbed by the thyroid gland from the bloodstream, providing insights into how the gland is functioning. An increased uptake is indicative of hyperthyroidism, especially in conditions like Graves' disease, whereas a lower uptake might suggest thyroiditis or exogenous sources of hyperthyroidism.

Thyroid Scan: A thyroid scan usually accompanies the RAIU test and involves imaging the thyroid gland after the administration of a radioactive substance. This scan provides a visual representation of the thyroid gland's size, shape, and activity, showing hot or cold nodules, which indicate their functioning status.

Ultrasound of the Thyroid: This non-invasive technique uses sound waves to create images of the thyroid gland and can detect the presence of nodules, cysts, or overall gland enlargement. Doppler ultrasound can assess blood flow, which might be increased in hyperthyroidism. It's particularly valuable for evaluating the physical characteristics of thyroid nodules and guiding fine-needle aspiration biopsies.

Fine-Needle Aspiration Biopsy: This procedure is often performed when a nodule is detected to rule out thyroid cancer, which is rare in hyperthyroidism but still a crucial consideration. A small needle is used to extract cells from the thyroid nodule for cytological examination.

Additional Considerations in Diagnosis

Physical Examination: A comprehensive physical exam includes looking for signs of hyperthyroidism such as a smooth, rapid pulse, tremors, warm, moist skin, and eye changes. A goiter or nodules might be palpable in the neck area. The physician will also look for signs of Graves' ophthalmopathy, including protruding eyes, swelling, or redness.

Medical and Family History: Detailed discussions about the patient's personal and family medical history can reveal risk factors or a genetic predisposition for thyroid disorders. Understanding any history of autoimmune diseases, previous head and neck irradiation, or recent iodine exposure is also critical.

Symptom Assessment: The doctor will assess symptoms that might suggest hyperthyroidism, including unintentional weight loss, increased appetite, heat intolerance, increased sweating, palpitations, anxiety, and changes in menstrual patterns in women.

The diagnostic process for hyperthyroidism is thorough, involving the integration of clinical findings, blood tests, and imaging results. Each diagnostic method provides different insights into the thyroid's function and health, contributing to a holistic understanding of the patient's condition. Given the variety of hyperthyroidism causes and presentations, a detailed and patient-specific approach is essential. Regular monitoring and follow-up are crucial, particularly to evaluate the effectiveness of treatment and make necessary adjustments. With accurate diagnosis and appropriate management, most individuals with hyperthyroidism can lead healthy and active lives.

Managing Hyperthyroidism

Managing hyperthyroidism, a condition characterized by the thyroid gland producing excess hormones, requires a comprehensive approach, involving medication, and in some cases, surgical or other non-surgical interventions. The treatment plan is typically tailored to the individual's specific condition, age, overall health, and personal preferences.

Medication Options

Antithyroid Drugs

Methimazole (Tapazole)

Mechanism of Action: Methimazole inhibits the synthesis of thyroid hormones by blocking the thyroid peroxidase enzyme, which is crucial in the iodination of thyroglobulin and subsequent thyroid hormone production.

Dosage and Administration: Initial dosing can be high, ranging from 10 to 40 mg daily, depending on the severity of hyperthyroidism. It's typically reduced once the patient achieves a euthyroid state. It can be given once daily due to its longer half-life.

Side Effects: Common side effects include minor rash and gastrointestinal upset. Serious but rare side effects include agranulocytosis (a significant decrease in white blood cell count) and hepatotoxicity. Regular monitoring of complete blood count and liver function tests is recommended.

Special Considerations: It is preferred in most non-pregnant adults. In pregnancy, its use is limited to the second and third trimesters due to teratogenic risks in the first trimester.

Propylthiouracil (PTU)

Mechanism of Action: PTU inhibits thyroid hormone synthesis similar to Methimazole. Additionally, it blocks the conversion of T4 to T3 in peripheral tissues.

Dosage: Requires multiple daily dosing, typically in the range of 100-600 mg per day, divided into two or three doses due to its shorter half-life.

Side Effects: Includes rash, arthralgia, and gastrointestinal disturbances. Hepatotoxicity is a serious concern, more common than with Methimazole. Agranulocytosis, although rare, is also a potential risk.

Special Considerations: Used during the first trimester of pregnancy and in managing thyroid storm due to its ability to block peripheral T4 to T3 conversion.

Beta-Blockers

Propranolol, Atenolol, Metoprolol

Purpose: Beta-blockers are prescribed to manage cardiovascular symptoms associated with hyperthyroidism, including palpitations, tremors, and anxiety.

Mechanism of Action: They inhibit the effects of adrenaline and noradrenaline on the heart and other tissues, thereby controlling heart rate, blood pressure, and tremors.

Dosage and Administration: The choice of beta-blocker and its dosage depend on the patient's cardiovascular status and specific symptoms. For example, Propranolol can be started at a dose of 10-40 mg every 6-8 hours, tailored based on the response and tolerance.

Considerations: They do not alter thyroid hormone levels but are crucial for symptom control, especially during the initial phase of treatment.

Iodine Solutions

Lugol's Solution, Potassium Iodide (SSKI)

Usage: Employed in preparing the thyroid gland for surgery and managing thyroid storm.

Mechanism of Action: High doses of iodine inhibit thyroid hormone synthesis and release, reducing the gland's size and vascularity.

Administration: Generally administered orally, the duration of treatment is short-term, often a week or two before surgery.

Monitoring and Long-term Management

Thyroid Function Tests: Regular monitoring of TSH, Free T4, and T3 is necessary to adjust medication dosages and assess the effectiveness of treatment.

Patient Education: It's vital to educate patients about recognizing symptoms indicative of potential side effects, especially those related to agranulocytosis or liver dysfunction.

Treatment Duration: Antithyroid medications are typically used for 12-18 months before attempting to taper or discontinue them. Some patients may require longer treatment or even lifelong therapy.

Special Considerations

Pregnancy and Lactation: Managing hyperthyroidism in pregnancy requires balancing the benefits and risks of medications. Methimazole is preferred in the second and third trimesters, while PTU is used during the first trimester and in thyroid storm.

Elderly Patients: In older patients, the management of hyperthyroidism must be approached cautiously, considering comorbid conditions and the increased risk of adverse effects.

Effective management of hyperthyroidism with medications requires a personalized approach, considering the patient's specific condition, response to treatment, and potential side effects. This often necessitates regular and open communication with healthcare providers, including endocrinologists, to ensure optimal treatment outcomes. Adjustments to the treatment plan may be necessary over time, based on the patient's response, changes in thyroid function, and any side effects experienced.

Surgical Treatments

Surgical treatment for hyperthyroidism, primarily involving thyroidectomy, is a crucial option in cases where medication and radioactive iodine therapy are not suitable or have failed to yield the desired results. The decision to opt for surgery is significant and depends on various factors, including the cause of hyperthyroidism, the size of the thyroid gland, the presence of nodules, and the patient's overall health and preferences.

There are two main types of thyroidectomy: total thyroidectomy, which involves the removal of the entire thyroid gland, and partial thyroidectomy, also known as subtotal thyroidectomy, where only part of the gland is removed.

Total thyroidectomy is often indicated in patients with Graves' disease, particularly those with severe ophthalmopathy, large goiters causing obstructive symptoms, or when there's a suspicion of thyroid cancer. This approach requires the patient to take lifelong thyroid hormone replacement therapy since the body's natural hormone production is halted. Partial thyroidectomy may be preferred in less severe cases of hyperthyroidism, such as when the condition is caused by a single overactive nodule. This surgery might allow for some thyroid function post-operation, reducing the likelihood of needing lifelong hormone therapy, though there's a risk of recurrence of hyperthyroidism.

The preoperative evaluation for thyroid surgery is comprehensive. It includes an assessment of vocal cord function to ensure they are not compromised, as they could be affected during surgery due to the proximity of the recurrent laryngeal nerves to the thyroid gland. In addition, thorough thyroid function tests and imaging studies, such as ultrasound or CT scans, are conducted to assess the size and nature of the thyroid gland and any nodules. Patients are also thoroughly counseled about the benefits, risks, and potential need for lifelong hormone replacement therapy post-surgery.

The surgical procedure is performed under general anesthesia. An incision is made in the neck to access the thyroid gland. Surgeons carefully remove the thyroid tissue, taking care to avoid damaging the parathyroid glands, which regulate calcium levels in the body, and preserve the recurrent laryngeal nerves, which are essential for voice. In some cases, intraoperative monitoring techniques are employed to minimize the risk of nerve damage.

Risks and complications associated with thyroid surgery include hypoparathyroidism, which can lead to a significant drop in calcium levels and requires treatment with calcium and vitamin D supplements. Damage to the recurrent laryngeal nerve can result in voice changes or hoarseness. Like any major surgery, there are also risks of hemorrhage, infection, and in rare cases, a thyroid storm, which is a sudden and severe increase in thyroid hormones. To mitigate these risks, patients are often medically stabilized before surgery.

Postoperative care involves monitoring calcium levels, especially after total thyroidectomy, to manage potential hypocalcemia. Patients who undergo total thyroidectomy require lifelong hormone replacement therapy with levothyroxine to maintain normal thyroid hormone levels. The dosage is tailored based on regular blood tests. Recovery includes monitoring for any changes in voice, pain or discomfort in the neck, and signs of infection or hematoma at the surgical site.

Special considerations are taken for pregnant women, where surgery might be preferred when antithyroid drugs are contraindicated or ineffective. Pediatric patients also require special attention due to their smaller anatomy and the long-term implications of thyroid removal.

Surgical treatment of hyperthyroidism, while definitive, requires careful patient selection, skilled surgical execution, and thorough postoperative management. Patients need to be well-informed about the procedure, its risks, and the lifestyle changes that may follow, including the possibility of lifelong hormone replacement therapy. Regular medical follow-up is essential to monitor for potential complications and adjust hormone therapy as needed.

Non-Surgical Treatments

Non-surgical treatments for hyperthyroidism, particularly Radioactive Iodine Therapy (RAI) and Ethanol Ablation Therapy provide effective alternatives to surgical intervention, especially for specific patient groups or types of hyperthyroidism.

Radioactive Iodine Therapy (RAI) is a cornerstone treatment, particularly effective for conditions like Graves' disease, toxic multinodular goiter, and toxic adenomas. This therapy involves orally administering I-131, a radioactive isotope of iodine. Since the thyroid gland naturally accumulates iodine to produce thyroid hormones, introducing it in a radioactive form leads to selective destruction of thyroid cells, thereby reducing the gland's hormone-producing capacity.

The procedure is simple, requiring patients to ingest RAI in capsule or liquid form. It's an outpatient procedure, but patients are advised to follow radiation safety precautions post-treatment. These include avoiding close physical contact, especially with vulnerable groups like children and pregnant women, and practicing good hygiene to minimize radiation exposure to others. The therapeutic effect of RAI might take weeks to months to fully manifest, and a common long-term outcome is hypothyroidism, necessitating lifelong thyroid hormone replacement therapy. Regular follow-up appointments, including thyroid function tests, are essential to monitor the effectiveness of the therapy and manage hormone replacement.

Ethanol Ablation Therapy is another non-surgical option, primarily used for benign autonomously functioning thyroid nodules and cystic nodules. It's particularly beneficial for patients not suited for surgery or RAI, such as those with smaller, localized thyroid nodules. The treatment is performed under local anesthesia and guided by ultrasound. A fine needle is used to inject ethanol directly into the thyroid nodules, causing cellular dehydration and necrosis within the nodules, thereby reducing their size and activity. The procedure may need repetition, depending on the nodules' size and response. Side effects can include transient pain or discomfort and, rarely, local inflammation or nerve damage. Post-treatment care involves ultrasound monitoring to assess the response and determine the need for additional sessions. Regular thyroid function tests ensure the overall thyroid status remains stable.

Both RAI and Ethanol Ablation Therapy are significant non-surgical options for managing hyperthyroidism, each with its suitability, effectiveness, and follow-up requirements. The choice between these therapies depends on various factors, including the underlying cause of hyperthyroidism, the patient's overall health, personal preferences, and specific characteristics of the thyroid gland. Careful patient selection, thorough pre-treatment evaluation, and counseling are crucial. Continuous monitoring and follow-up care are integral to assessing treatment efficacy and managing any resultant conditions, such as hypothyroidism post-RAI, ensuring optimal patient outcomes.

Chapter Four: Other Thyroid Conditions

In this chapter, we delve into a spectrum of thyroid-related disorders beyond the commonly discussed hyperthyroidism and hypothyroidism. This chapter offers an in-depth exploration of Thyroid Nodules and Goiter, conditions characterized by abnormal growths and enlargement of the thyroid gland, respectively. We then navigate through the complexities of Thyroiditis and Its Variants, including Hashimoto's thyroiditis and postpartum thyroiditis, which illustrate the thyroid's vulnerability to inflammatory processes.

The critical and often challenging topic of Thyroid Cancer is addressed, providing insights into its diagnosis, treatment, and management. Finally, the chapter concludes with a section on Rare Thyroid Disorders, shedding light on lesser-known yet significant thyroid conditions. Each section combines current medical understanding with practical insights, ensuring a comprehensive overview of these varied thyroid pathologies.

Thyroid Nodules and Goiter

Thyroid nodules and goiter are significant conditions affecting the thyroid gland, each presenting unique diagnostic and management challenges.

Thyroid Nodules are localized enlargements within the thyroid gland, varying in size and nature. They can develop from an overgrowth of normal thyroid tissue, from cyst formation, or as a result of thyroid inflammation. Risk factors for developing thyroid nodules include age (more common in older adults), a family history of thyroid disease, iodine deficiency, and exposure to radiation, particularly during childhood.

These nodules can be benign, such as colloid nodules, follicular adenomas, and cysts, or malignant, indicating thyroid cancer. Functionally, they can be classified as hyperfunctioning (producing excess thyroid hormones), non-functioning, or hypo-functioning, affecting the overall thyroid hormone balance in the body. Diagnosis begins with a physical examination where the doctor may palpate the neck to detect nodules.

Blood tests for thyroid function, including TSH, Free T4, and Free T3 levels, help assess the activity of the thyroid gland. Ultrasound is a crucial tool in evaluating the size, number, and characteristics of the nodules – distinguishing between solid and cystic nodules. For nodules that are suspicious in nature or exceed a certain size, Fine-Needle Aspiration Biopsy (FNAB) is performed. This procedure involves extracting cells from the nodule using a fine needle, which are then examined under a microscope to assess the risk of cancer.

The management of thyroid nodules depends significantly on their nature. Benign nodules are often managed with regular monitoring, including periodic ultrasounds and thyroid function tests. If benign nodules grow large, cause compressive symptoms like difficulty swallowing or breathing, or raise cosmetic concerns, treatment options may include surgical removal or thyroid hormone suppression therapy. This therapy aims to suppress TSH with levothyroxine, potentially reducing nodule growth.

Malignant nodules, on the other hand, are typically managed with a more aggressive approach. This usually involves surgery – partial or total thyroidectomy – often followed by radioactive iodine therapy to destroy any remaining cancerous tissue. Post-surgical management includes lifelong thyroid hormone replacement therapy for patients undergoing total thyroidectomy.

Goiter refers to a generalized enlargement of the thyroid gland and can manifest in various forms. The causes of goiters include iodine deficiency (the most common cause worldwide), Hashimoto's thyroiditis (an autoimmune condition leading to chronic thyroid inflammation), Graves' disease (where the thyroid is diffusely overactive), multinodular goiter, certain medications that affect thyroid function, and hormonal changes (such as during pregnancy). In some cases, goiters can also develop due to thyroid cancer.

Goiters can be classified as diffuse, involving a uniform enlargement of the thyroid, or nodular, featuring distinct lumps within the gland. They are also categorized based on thyroid function: euthyroid goiters (with normal thyroid function), hyperthyroid goiters (associated with overactive thyroid function), or hypothyroid goiters (associated with underactive thyroid function).

The diagnosis of goiter starts with a physical examination, where the doctor assesses the size and texture of the thyroid gland. Thyroid function tests are then performed to determine if the goiter is associated with hypo- or hyperthyroidism. Ultrasound is used to assess the size and nature of the goiter, and in certain cases, a radioiodine scan is conducted to provide detailed information about thyroid function and structure.

Management of goiter varies based on its cause and associated thyroid function. Euthyroid goiters are often monitored regularly without immediate intervention, but surgery or radioactive iodine treatment may be considered if the goiter causes compressive symptoms (such as difficulty swallowing or breathing) or for cosmetic reasons. Hyperthyroid goiters may require antithyroid drugs, radioactive iodine therapy, or surgical intervention, depending on the underlying cause and severity. Hypothyroid goiters are typically managed with thyroid hormone replacement therapy to restore normal thyroid function.

In managing both thyroid nodules and goiter, the approach is personalized, often requiring adjustments based on the patient's response and any changes in the condition. Regular follow-up is critical for monitoring the condition, managing symptoms, and adjusting treatment as necessary. In cases where malignancy is suspected or confirmed, a more aggressive treatment approach is warranted, including consideration for surgery and possible radioactive iodine therapy. Regular medical follow-ups are crucial to monitor for potential complications or recurrence of hyperthyroidism.

Thyroiditis and Its Variants

Thyroiditis, characterized by inflammation of the thyroid gland, encompasses several distinct disorders, each with unique etiological factors, clinical presentations, and management approaches.

Hashimoto's Thyroiditis (Chronic Lymphocytic Thyroiditis) is an autoimmune disorder and the most common type of thyroiditis. In this condition, the immune system mistakenly attacks thyroid tissue, leading to chronic inflammation and often resulting in hypothyroidism. Patients with Hashimoto's thyroiditis typically experience symptoms associated with an underactive thyroid, including fatigue, weight gain, constipation, dry skin, hair loss, cold intolerance, and depression. Some may initially go through a phase of hyperthyroidism, known as Hashitoxicosis, due to the release of thyroid hormones from the damaged thyroid cells.

Diagnostically, Hashimoto's thyroiditis is identified by elevated levels of thyroid antibodies (anti-thyroid peroxidase and anti-thyroglobulin antibodies) in the blood. Thyroid function tests often show reduced levels of thyroid hormones, and ultrasound imaging of the gland may reveal a characteristic heterogeneous echotexture. Management typically involves long-term thyroid hormone replacement therapy with levothyroxine. The dosage is adjusted based on regular monitoring of thyroid-stimulating hormonc (TSH) levels to ensure optimal thyroid function.

De Quervain's Thyroiditis (Subacute Thyroiditis) is often triggered by a viral infection and is characterized by painful inflammation of the thyroid gland. This condition typically follows an upper respiratory infection and presents with a tender, swollen thyroid gland, fever, malaise, and symptoms indicative of hyperthyroidism. These symptoms are usually transient and are followed by a hypothyroid phase before the thyroid function typically returns to normal.

Diagnostic tests reveal elevated erythrocyte sedimentation rate (ESR) and C-reactive protein (CRP) levels, indicative of inflammation. Thyroid function tests during the course of the disease show transient hyperthyroidism followed by hypothyroidism. Treatment primarily focuses on managing pain and inflammation using non-steroidal anti-inflammatory drugs (NSAIDs) or corticosteroids. Beta-blockers may be prescribed to control symptoms of hyperthyroidism. The condition generally resolves on its own; however, regular monitoring of thyroid function is crucial to guide the need for any further intervention.

Silent Thyroiditis (Painless Thyroiditis), an autoimmune condition often seen in postpartum women, is similar to Hashimoto's thyroiditis but is usually of a transient nature. Patients typically experience a brief period of hyperthyroidism, followed by hypothyroidism, and then a return to normal thyroid function, usually without significant pain or tenderness in the thyroid gland. Management involves symptom control during both the hyperthyroid and hypothyroid phases. Beta-blockers are utilized to alleviate hyperthyroid symptoms, and temporary thyroid hormone replacement may be required during the hypothyroid phase.

Postpartum Thyroiditis is a specific form of silent thyroiditis that occurs in women after childbirth. It follows a similar pattern, starting with a phase of hyperthyroidism followed by hypothyroidism. The symptoms can include fatigue, mood swings, and weight changes. The treatment for postpartum thyroiditis is symptomatic and similar to that for silent thyroiditis. While most women recover normal thyroid function, a proportion may develop permanent hypothyroidism.

Acute Infectious Thyroiditis is a rare but severe form of thyroiditis caused by a bacterial infection. It is often associated with a compromised immune system or pre-existing thyroid conditions. Symptoms include severe neck pain and swelling, fever, and general signs of infection, along with thyroid dysfunction symptoms. The treatment primarily involves administering antibiotics to treat the underlying bacterial infection. Surgical drainage may become necessary when an abscess arises.

Riedel's Thyroiditis is an extremely rare, chronic form characterized by extensive fibrosis replacing normal thyroid tissue, leading to a hard, painless enlargement of the thyroid gland. This can cause compressive symptoms in the neck. Patients may also develop hypothyroidism due to the destruction of thyroid tissue. The treatment for Riedel's thyroiditis includes thyroid hormone replacement therapy for managing hypothyroidism. Corticosteroids or other immunosuppressive agents are used to reduce inflammation. In cases where the fibrosis causes significant compression of neck structures, surgical intervention might be necessary to relieve the symptoms.

The management of thyroiditis, regardless of the specific type, requires a comprehensive approach that addresses both the acute and long-term aspects of the disease. Regular monitoring of thyroid function is essential in all types of thyroiditis to assess the need for and response to treatment. Symptom management, particularly in the acute phases of thyroiditis, is important. This can include pain management and control of thyroid hormone levels with medication, and in some cases, addressing the underlying cause, such as infection.

In conditions like Hashimoto's thyroiditis, which often leads to permanent hypothyroidism, lifelong thyroid hormone replacement therapy is necessary. For conditions with a transient course, such as De Quervain's or silent thyroiditis, treatment is more focused on symptom relief and monitoring until thyroid function normalizes. Regular follow-up and thyroid function monitoring are essential to ensure appropriate treatment and manage the long-term implications of these conditions.

Thyroid Cancer

Thyroid cancer, originating from the cells of the thyroid gland, presents in various forms, each with distinct risk factors, diagnostic methods, treatment modalities, and prognoses. Understanding the nuances of these cancer types is crucial for effective management and patient care.

Papillary Thyroid Cancer (PTC) is the most prevalent type of thyroid cancer. It typically arises from the follicular cells of the thyroid and is known for its slow growth. PTC frequently presents as a painless mass in the neck and has a tendency to spread to lymph nodes. Key risk factors include exposure to radiation, especially during childhood, a family history of thyroid cancer, and specific genetic mutations. PTC is more common in women and typically affects patients in their 30s and 40s.

Follicular Thyroid Cancer (FTC), while also originating from follicular cells, is more aggressive than PTC. It has a higher propensity for hematogenous spread, particularly to the lungs and bones. FTC shares similar risk factors with PTC, including radiation exposure and genetic predispositions, with an increased incidence in iodine-deficient areas.

Medullary Thyroid Cancer (MTC) develops from the parafollicular C cells of the thyroid, responsible for producing calcitonin. MTC is unique for its secretion of calcitonin, which serves as a diagnostic and monitoring marker. About 25% of MTC cases are familial, related to mutations in the RET gene, seen in conditions like multiple endocrine neoplasia (MEN) syndromes. Sporadic MTC typically occurs in older adults.

Anaplastic Thyroid Cancer (ATC) is a rare, extremely aggressive form of thyroid cancer. It is known for its rapid growth and poor response to traditional treatments, often presenting in advanced stages. Risk factors for ATC include advanced age and a history of goiter or long-standing thyroid disease.

The diagnosis of thyroid cancer usually begins with the detection of a nodule during a physical examination or incidentally on imaging for unrelated reasons. Blood tests assess thyroid function, and specifically for MTC, calcitonin levels are measured. Ultrasound examination of the thyroid is critical in evaluating nodules and guiding fine-needle aspiration biopsies. FNAB is the definitive diagnostic tool, involving the extraction of cells from the thyroid nodule for cytological examination. Advanced imaging techniques, such as CT scans, MRI, and PET scans, are employed to assess the extent of the disease, especially in more advanced cases.

Treatment typically involves surgical intervention, with the extent of surgery (total thyroidectomy versus lobectomy) determined based on the cancer type, stage, and patient factors. Radioactive Iodine Therapy (RAI) is commonly used postoperatively for PTC and FTC to ablate residual thyroid tissue and address metastatic disease. Following surgery, thyroid hormone therapy is initiated to replace hormones and suppress TSH, reducing the risk of recurrence. In the case of ATC and other advanced thyroid cancers, external beam radiation therapy and chemotherapy are considered. Targeted therapy is increasingly employed for advanced or recurrent thyroid cancers that do not respond to conventional treatments.

The prognosis for thyroid cancer varies depending on the type. PTC and FTC generally have an excellent prognosis, particularly when detected early and treated appropriately. The prognosis for MTC is more variable and often depends on the stage at diagnosis and the presence of genetic mutations. ATC, due to its aggressive nature, typically has a poor prognosis, with treatment focusing on palliative care to improve quality of life.

Management of thyroid cancer involves a multidisciplinary team approach, incorporating the expertise of endocrinologists, oncologists, surgeons, and radiologists. Lifelong monitoring is essential due to the potential for recurrence, particularly in more aggressive types. Recent advances in genetic research and targeted therapies are improving outcomes for patients with advanced thyroid cancers. Early detection, careful monitoring of thyroid nodules, and prompt, appropriate intervention remain key to successful treatment outcomes. Regular follow-up post-treatment is crucial for managing potential complications and detecting any recurrence at an early, more treatable stage.

Rare Thyroid Disorders

Rare thyroid disorders, while uncommon, present unique challenges in terms of diagnosis, treatment, and management. Each condition requires a tailored approach due to its specific characteristics.

Thyroid Dysgenesis is a congenital anomaly where the thyroid gland is either absent, ectopically located, or underdeveloped. It's a significant cause of congenital hypothyroidism. Affected newborns may exhibit symptoms like prolonged jaundice, feeding difficulties, constipation, and poor muscle tone. These symptoms are critical to identify early to prevent developmental delays. Diagnosis typically follows abnormal results from newborn thyroid screening tests, with subsequent imaging like ultrasound or scintigraphy confirming the gland's abnormality. Treatment involves immediate and lifelong thyroid hormone replacement to support normal growth and development, with regular monitoring to adjust the hormone dosage as the child grows.

Thyroid Hemangioma is a rare, benign vascular tumor within the thyroid gland. These tumors can vary in size and are often asymptomatic. However, larger hemangiomas may cause neck swelling, discomfort, or even hyperthyroidism due to increased vascularity. Diagnosis is usually incidental during imaging studies for unrelated issues. Ultrasound, CT, or MRI can help in diagnosing, and fine-needle aspiration biopsy is sometimes necessary for differentiation from other thyroid masses. Treatment is generally conservative, but surgical removal may be needed for large hemangiomas causing symptoms. Regular monitoring is crucial to track any changes in size or symptomatology.

Pendred Syndrome, a genetic disorder, leads to sensorineural hearing loss and thyroid dysfunction. It's linked to mutations in the SLC26A4 gene affecting iodine metabolism. The syndrome presents with hearing impairment from early childhood and goiter development during adolescence or adulthood. Diagnosis is based on clinical symptoms, genetic testing for SLC26A4 mutations, and thyroid imaging. Management focuses on addressing hearing loss, often requiring hearing aids or cochlear implants, and monitoring thyroid function and goiter development. Thyroid hormone replacement therapy may be necessary for those who develop hypothyroidism.

Thyroid Teratoma is an extremely rare tumor, generally benign, comprising various tissue types. These tumors are more aggressive in adults than in children. Symptoms usually include a palpable neck mass, and in some cases, there may be signs of hyperthyroidism. Imaging techniques like ultrasound and MRI are employed for diagnosis, and a biopsy is conducted to confirm the nature of the tumor and rule out malignancy. The primary treatment is surgical excision, with careful post-surgical follow-up essential to monitor for recurrence or other complications.

The management of these rare thyroid conditions often involves a multidisciplinary team, including endocrinologists, pediatricians, surgeons, and geneticists. Early diagnosis and intervention are particularly crucial in congenital conditions like thyroid dysgenesis and Pendred syndrome to prevent long-term complications and ensure optimal growth and development. Lifelong monitoring and individualized treatment plans are key for managing these disorders effectively, highlighting the importance of specialized care and regular follow-up in rare thyroid disorders.

Chapter Five: Lifestyle and Thyroid Health

Here, we explore the vital role that daily habits and choices play in the functioning and well-being of the thyroid gland. Delving into Diet and Nutrition, we uncover how certain foods and nutrients directly influence thyroid health. We then navigate through the impacts of Exercise and Physical Activity, understanding their importance in maintaining optimal thyroid function.

The chapter also addresses the often-overlooked connection between the thyroid and mental well-being, examining how Stress, Sleep, and Mental Health are intricately linked to thyroid health. Lastly, we venture into the realm of Integrative and Alternative Therapies, discussing how these approaches can complement traditional medical treatments and support overall thyroid health.

Diet and Nutrition

The intricate relationship between diet, nutrition, and thyroid health is increasingly recognized as a vital aspect of managing thyroid function. A well-considered diet can significantly support the thyroid, a gland crucial for metabolic regulation, growth, and development.

Iodine's Role in Thyroid Health

Iodine is essential for the synthesis of thyroid hormones, thyroxine (T4), and triiodothyronine (T3), which regulate numerous physiological processes. The body cannot produce iodine, necessitating its intake through diet. Natural sources include seaweed, fish, dairy products, and iodized salt. While iodine deficiency can lead to hypothyroidism and goiter, excess iodine intake can also trigger thyroid dysfunction, making a balanced intake critical. Pregnant and breastfeeding women need to be particularly mindful of their iodine intake due to increased demands for thyroid hormone production during these stages.

Selenium's Contribution to Thyroid Function

Selenium, a trace element, is integral to the thyroid gland's health. It contributes to the production and metabolism of thyroid hormones and offers protection against oxidative damage within the thyroid gland. Brazil nuts are an exceptionally rich source of selenium, but their consumption should be moderated due to the risk of selenium toxicity. Other sources like fish, poultry, and seeds provide selenium in safer amounts. Selenium's role is particularly crucial in the enzymatic conversion of T4 into its active form, T3, making it an indispensable nutrient for optimal thyroid function.

Zinc and Thyroid Hormone Synthesis

Zinc is another mineral that plays a significant role in thyroid hormone synthesis and conversion. Foods rich in zinc, such as oysters, red meat, poultry, nuts, and legumes, can help maintain healthy thyroid function. Zinc deficiencies can manifest as hypothyroidism symptoms, and supplementation can be beneficial, especially in individuals with compromised thyroid function.

Fiber for Digestive Health in Thyroid Disorders

Maintaining a healthy digestive system is particularly important for those with thyroid disorders. A diet rich in fiber aids in digestion and helps alleviate constipation, a common symptom of hypothyroidism. Sources of dietary fiber include whole grains, legumes, fruits, and vegetables. Fiber also plays a role in maintaining a healthy weight, which can be challenging for those with thyroid disorders.

Antioxidants to Combat Oxidative Stress

The thyroid gland is susceptible to oxidative stress, which can exacerbate thyroid dysfunction. Consuming antioxidant-rich foods like berries, nuts, green leafy vegetables, and seeds can help mitigate this risk. These foods provide a natural defense against oxidative damage and support overall thyroid health.

The Importance of Iron in Thyroid Health

Iron deficiency, which can impair thyroid hormone metabolism, is commonly seen in individuals with hypothyroidism. Adequate iron intake through diet or supplementation is necessary to support thyroid function. Red meat, legumes, fortified cereals, and green leafy vegetables are good sources of iron.

Vitamin D and Immune Regulation

Vitamin D plays a role in immune regulation and has been linked to a higher risk of autoimmune thyroid diseases. Adequate vitamin D levels, achievable through sun exposure, diet, and supplementation, are important for maintaining immune and thyroid health. Egg yolks, dairy products with added fortification, and fatty fish are food sources of vitamin D.

Vitamin B12 for Metabolic Function

Vitamin B12 is essential for metabolic processes and is often found to be deficient in individuals with thyroid dysfunction. Regular intake of B12, through sources such as meat, fish, dairy products, and fortified foods, or via supplementation, is important, particularly for those on thyroid medications.

Additional Dietary Considerations

Gluten and Thyroid Function: Gluten sensitivity can exacerbate autoimmune responses in susceptible individuals, particularly those with Hashimoto's thyroiditis. A gluten-free diet may offer benefits in these cases.

Goitrogens and Thyroid Function: Certain foods contain goitrogens, which may interfere with thyroid hormone production. Cruciferous vegetables, soy products, and certain types of millet fall into this category. Cooking these foods typically reduces their goitrogenic effect.

Processed Foods and Sugars: Limiting intake of processed and high-sugar foods is advised as these can lead to weight gain and metabolic disturbances, worsening symptoms of thyroid disorders.

For individuals with thyroid conditions, consulting with healthcare professionals, including dietitians, is essential to devise a diet plan that supports thyroid health. This includes regular monitoring of thyroid function and nutritional status to guide dietary adjustments, ensuring optimal health outcomes. Diet and nutrition are powerful tools in managing thyroid health, emphasizing the importance of a well-balanced, nutrient-rich diet.

Exercise and Physical Activity

The role of exercise and physical activity in maintaining thyroid health is multifaceted and significant, especially for those managing thyroid disorders. A deeper understanding of how different types of exercise can benefit thyroid function, as well as considerations for safe and effective physical activity, is crucial.

Expanded Insights into Aerobic Exercises

Aerobic exercises, also known as cardio workouts, are critical for cardiovascular health and play a vital role in managing symptoms associated with thyroid disorders. These exercises include activities like brisk walking, jogging, swimming, cycling, and group aerobic classes. For individuals with thyroid conditions, particularly hypothyroidism, aerobic exercises can help combat the sluggish metabolism and weight gain that are often symptomatic of the disorder.

Regular aerobic activity improves cardiovascular fitness, boosts metabolism, and aids in weight control. It's recommended that adults engage in at least 150 minutes of moderate-intensity aerobic activity or 75 minutes of vigorous activity each week, according to guidelines set by health organizations. However, it's important for individuals with thyroid disorders to gradually build up their endurance and intensity to avoid overexertion, which can exacerbate symptoms.

Strength Training for Thyroid Health

Strength or resistance training is a valuable component of an exercise regimen for thyroid health. Building muscle mass through activities like weight lifting, resistance band exercises, and bodyweight exercises (such as push-ups, squats, and lunges) helps boost the body's metabolism. This is particularly beneficial for those with hypothyroidism, who often experience a reduced metabolic rate.

Muscle tissue burns more calories at rest compared to fat tissue, thus aiding in weight management and overall energy levels. Engaging in strength training exercises at least twice a week is advised, targeting all major muscle groups. For individuals with thyroid disorders, it's important to start with lower weights or resistance levels and gradually increase them to prevent muscle strain and fatigue.

The Benefits of Yoga and Flexibility Exercises

Yoga and flexibility exercises offer unique benefits for individuals with thyroid disorders. Specific yoga poses, such as the shoulder stand or fish pose, are believed to stimulate the thyroid gland and may help in regulating thyroid function. The practice of yoga incorporates deep breathing and meditative techniques that contribute to stress reduction and mental well-being, both of which are crucial for individuals with thyroid issues.

Chronic stress can have adverse effects on thyroid function, making relaxation and stress-management techniques important. In addition, yoga and stretching exercises improve flexibility, balance, and body awareness, which can enhance overall physical fitness and well-being.

Low-Impact Exercises for Joint Health and Thyroid Function

For those experiencing joint pain or discomfort, common in thyroid disorders, low-impact exercises such as swimming, water aerobics, or stationary cycling can be excellent alternatives. These activities provide the cardiovascular benefits of aerobic exercise without placing excessive strain on the joints. Low-impact exercises are particularly suitable for those who are overweight, elderly, or recovering from an injury, offering a safer option that still contributes to thyroid health.

Understanding the Impact on Thyroid Function and Hormone Levels

Regular physical activity positively influences thyroid function in several ways. Exercise stimulates the body's metabolism, aiding in the more efficient use of thyroid hormones. This is especially beneficial in hypothyroidism, where metabolic rates are typically reduced. Exercise also helps regulate the levels of stress hormones in the body, which, when elevated, can negatively impact thyroid function. Additionally, by aiding in weight management and improving metabolic rate, exercise can enhance the overall efficacy of thyroid hormones in the body. Improved cardiovascular fitness, increased energy levels, and enhanced mood from regular physical activity also contribute significantly to the quality of life for individuals with thyroid disorders.

In summary, incorporating a varied exercise regimen that includes aerobic workouts, strength training, yoga, and low-impact activities is highly beneficial for thyroid health. Individuals with thyroid conditions need to approach exercise with caution, starting slowly and gradually increasing intensity to avoid exacerbating symptoms. Regular consultation with healthcare providers and careful monitoring of thyroid function and overall health are important to ensure that the exercise plan is appropriate and effective for individual needs. Regular physical activity, tailored to one's capabilities and health status, is an integral part of managing thyroid health and enhancing overall well-being.

Stress, Sleep, and Mental Health

The intricate interplay between stress, sleep, mental health, and thyroid function is a crucial aspect of managing thyroid health.

Stress, in particular, has a profound impact on thyroid function. Chronic stress activates the hypothalamic-pituitary-adrenal (HPA) axis, leading to elevated cortisol levels. This increase in the body's primary stress hormone can suppress thyroid-stimulating hormone (TSH) and inhibit the conversion of Thyroxine (T4) to Triiodothyronine (T3), leading to symptoms of hypothyroidism such as fatigue, weight gain, and depression.

Additionally, stress can exacerbate autoimmune thyroid conditions like Hashimoto's thyroiditis and Graves' disease. In these cases, stress-induced alterations in immune function can intensify the autoimmune attack on the thyroid gland, leading to inflammation and altered thyroid function. Furthermore, in individuals with pre-existing thyroid conditions, stress can amplify symptoms, making stress management an essential component of comprehensive thyroid disorder treatment.

The role of sleep and mental well-being in thyroid health cannot be overstated. Quality sleep is vital for maintaining the body's circadian rhythms, which regulate the secretion of TSH. Disruptions in sleep patterns can lead to imbalances in thyroid hormones, exacerbating thyroid disorder symptoms. Additionally, adequate sleep is crucial for the body's recovery and hormonal balance. It helps in regulating stress hormones like cortisol, which can impact thyroid function.

The connection between mental well-being and thyroid function is also profound. There is a strong link between thyroid dysfunction and mood disorders. Hypothyroidism is commonly associated with depressive symptoms, while hyperthyroidism can be linked to anxiety and irritability. Addressing mental health is key in managing thyroid health. Thyroid imbalances can affect cognitive functions, such as memory and concentration. Therefore, improving mental health through stress management can help alleviate these cognitive symptoms.

Adopting a comprehensive approach to managing stress, sleep, and mental health is integral to maintaining thyroid health. Advanced stress management techniques, such as guided imagery, biofeedback, and cognitive restructuring, provide effective tools for coping with stressors and reducing their impact on thyroid health. Enhanced sleep hygiene practices, including developing a consistent sleep routine and optimizing the sleep environment, can significantly improve sleep quality.

Seeking support from psychologists, psychiatrists, or counselors is beneficial for those dealing with significant stress or mental health issues related to thyroid disorders. Therapeutic interventions like psychotherapy, group therapy, or medication management can offer substantial relief and support. Incorporating a variety of physical activities, including aerobic exercises, strength training, yoga, and tai chi, provides comprehensive benefits for stress reduction, mood improvement, and better sleep.

In summary, effectively managing stress, prioritizing sleep, and addressing mental health concerns are integral to maintaining thyroid health. Chronic stress can negatively impact thyroid function, while quality sleep and good mental health are essential for hormonal balance and effective management of thyroid disorder symptoms. Individuals with thyroid conditions should adopt a multidimensional approach to manage these aspects effectively. This approach includes lifestyle changes, therapeutic interventions, and regular consultations with healthcare professionals to ensure an integrated treatment plan.

Integrative and Alternative Therapies

Expanding on the integrative and alternative therapies for thyroid health, let's delve deeper into each approach, exploring their mechanisms, specific practices, benefits, and considerations. This detailed narrative will provide an extensive understanding of how these therapies can be effectively integrated into the management of thyroid disorders.

Integrative and alternative therapies for thyroid health encompass a broad spectrum of practices, offering a more holistic approach to complement conventional medical treatments. The cornerstone of this approach is nutritional therapy, emphasizing the importance of a balanced diet rich in essential nutrients for thyroid function. Iodine, crucial for the production of thyroid hormones, is abundantly found in seafood, dairy products, and iodized salt. Selenium and zinc, vital for thyroid hormone metabolism and immune function, are present in nuts, seeds, meats, and seafood. Additionally, vitamins like Vitamin D, often deficient in individuals with thyroid disorders, play a pivotal role in immune regulation and thyroid function. B-complex vitamins, particularly B12, are essential for energy metabolism and neurological function, often impaired in thyroid disorders.

Dietary patterns also have a significant impact on thyroid health. Anti-inflammatory diets, such as the Mediterranean diet, can benefit thyroid health by reducing systemic inflammation. For those with autoimmune thyroid conditions like Hashimoto's thyroiditis, a gluten-free diet may be recommended due to the potential link between gluten sensitivity and autoimmune reactions. However, it's crucial to approach dietary changes with balance and caution, avoiding restrictive diets that could lead to nutritional deficiencies.

Herbal medicine offers a range of options for supporting thyroid health. Adaptogenic herbs, including Ashwagandha, Rhodiola, and Holy Basil, are believed to modulate the body's stress response, potentially benefiting thyroid function by restoring hormonal balance and supporting the immune system. Guggul, an Ayurvedic herb, has been traditionally used for hypothyroidism, thought to enhance thyroid activity. However, the use of herbs requires careful consideration due to potential interactions with conventional thyroid medications and the risk of over or underconsumption of active compounds.

Acupuncture and Traditional Chinese Medicine (TCM) present a unique perspective on thyroid health, focusing on restoring energy balance and harmony within the body. Acupuncture, involving the insertion of fine needles into specific body points, is believed to stimulate the nervous system and affect the body's pain and stress responses. This may indirectly impact thyroid function by alleviating stress and promoting overall hormonal balance. TCM also encompasses a variety of herbal formulas, often personalized, aimed at correcting the specific imbalances identified in the individual, which are believed to influence thyroid health.

Mind-body practices, including yoga, meditation, Tai Chi, and Qi Gong, are increasingly recognized for their potential in managing thyroid disorders. These practices emphasize stress reduction, which is crucial given the impact of stress on both hyperthyroidism and hypothyroidism. Yoga, with specific asanas like the shoulder stand and fish pose, is thought to stimulate the thyroid gland directly. Meditation and relaxation techniques can help in managing the psychological and emotional challenges associated with thyroid disorders, improving overall well-being and potentially impacting thyroid health.

The efficacy of integrative and alternative therapies in managing thyroid health varies, with some approaches like nutritional therapy and stress reduction techniques having more substantial support in scientific literature. Personalized effectiveness is a key aspect, as individual responses to these therapies can differ significantly. Thus, it's essential for individuals to work closely with healthcare professionals to integrate these therapies into their overall treatment plan safely.

In integrating these therapies with conventional care, it's critical to maintain open communication with healthcare providers. Regular monitoring of thyroid function and medication interactions is necessary, as alternative therapies can influence hormone levels and medication efficacy. The choice of high-quality supplements and herbal products from reputable sources is paramount to ensure safety and efficacy.

In conclusion, integrative and alternative therapies offer a valuable and comprehensive approach to managing thyroid health, addressing not just the physical aspects of thyroid disorders but also the emotional and psychological components. While these therapies provide additional support and can enhance quality of life, they should be viewed as complementary to, not a replacement for, conventional medical treatments. A well-informed, cautious, and balanced approach, under the guidance of healthcare professionals, is essential for their effective and safe integration into thyroid health management.

Chapter Six: Navigating Thyroid Disorder Management

This chapter offers guidance on the importance of regular monitoring and testing, a crucial step for staying informed and proactive about your thyroid health. It delves into the nuances of adjusting to medication and treatment changes, highlighting the need for patience and adaptability in managing a dynamic condition. A significant focus is placed on coping with chronic illness, providing strategies for dealing with the physical, emotional, and psychological challenges of thyroid disorders.

Finally, the chapter empowers readers with tools for self-advocacy, emphasizing the importance of being an active participant in their healthcare journey. Through this chapter, readers will gain valuable insights and practical advice for navigating the complex path of thyroid disorder management.

Regular Monitoring and Testing

Regular monitoring and testing are pivotal in the effective management of thyroid disorders, serving as integral tools for diagnosing, guiding treatment, and ensuring long-term health stability. The dynamic nature of thyroid function, influenced by age, lifestyle changes, other health conditions, and medication interactions, necessitates a robust approach to ongoing assessment. Initially, when a thyroid disorder is diagnosed or when treatment begins, testing is frequent to fine-tune medication dosages. As treatment progresses and stabilizes, the frequency of these tests typically reduces, though it may vary with changes in symptoms or overall health status.

The primary test in thyroid health management is the Thyroid-Stimulating Hormone (TSH) test. TSH, produced by the pituitary gland, regulates the thyroid gland's production of thyroid hormones thyroxine (T4) and triiodothyronine (T3). TSH levels are inversely related to thyroid gland activity. Elevated TSH levels often indicate an underactive thyroid (hypothyroidism), where low thyroid hormone levels prompt the pituitary to produce more TSH. Conversely, low TSH levels can suggest an overactive thyroid (hyperthyroidism), where excess thyroid hormones suppress TSH production. The TSH test, therefore, is a crucial indicator of thyroid health and guides treatment adjustments.

In addition to TSH, Free T4 and Free T3 tests provide more specific insights into thyroid function. These tests measure the levels of unbound, active thyroid hormones circulating in the bloodstream. Free T4 and Free T3 are critical in evaluating the thyroid's direct output and metabolic effects on the body. Total T4 and T3 tests, measuring both bound and unbound hormones, can be beneficial in certain clinical situations, such as when protein-binding abnormalities are suspected.

Thyroid antibody tests, including Thyroid Peroxidase Antibodies (TPOAb), Thyroglobulin Antibodies (TgAb), and TSH Receptor Antibodies (TRAb), are essential for diagnosing autoimmune thyroid conditions. The presence and levels of these antibodies help in identifying conditions like Hashimoto's thyroiditis, characterized by TPOAb and TgAb, and Graves' disease, often associated with elevated TRAb. Monitoring these antibody levels over time can provide insight into the autoimmune process's activity and progression.

The frequency and timing of thyroid tests are tailored to individual needs. While more frequent testing is common in the initial stages of diagnosis and treatment, this typically decreases as a stable thyroid state is achieved. However, certain life stages, such as pregnancy, menopause, and significant aging, can significantly impact thyroid function and may require adjusted monitoring schedules.

Understanding and accurately interpreting thyroid test results is crucial for effective disease management. The interpretation of TSH, T4, and T3 levels must be done considering each patient's clinical context, including age, symptoms, and existing health conditions. Additionally, factors such as medications, supplements (notably biotin), and even the time of day can influence these hormone levels and should be considered when evaluating test results.

In summary, regular monitoring and testing form the cornerstone of thyroid disorder management. They provide valuable insights into the thyroid gland's functioning, enabling healthcare providers to make timely and effective treatment decisions. Patients play a vital role in this process, staying informed about their condition and understanding the implications of their test results. This collaborative approach ensures optimal management of thyroid health, adapting to changes over time and maintaining overall well-being.

Adjusting to Medication and Treatment Changes

Adjusting to medication and treatment changes is a critical component in the management of thyroid disorders. This process demands patients to be acutely attuned to their bodies and symptoms, as these are often the first indicators that adjustments might be necessary. For instance, changes in energy levels, weight, mood, and other physical symptoms like hair loss or changes in skin texture can signal an imbalance in thyroid hormones.

The emergence of new symptoms or the recurrence of previous ones, such as increased fatigue or depressive states, also suggests that the current treatment may need reevaluation. This vigilant monitoring of symptoms is essential for timely adjustments in medication and treatment. Regular thyroid function testing is a cornerstone in guiding these adjustments. Tests such as TSH, Free T4, and Free T3 are crucial in providing objective measures of thyroid function under the current treatment regimen.

Understanding these test results in the context of one's symptoms and overall health is vital. For example, even if TSH levels fall within the normal range, the dosage might still be suboptimal for some individuals, particularly if symptoms persist. It is important for patients to have a clear understanding of their lab values and to engage in discussions with their healthcare providers about how these numbers relate to their symptoms.

The dynamic nature of life means that lifestyle and physiological changes can significantly impact thyroid health and treatment. Dietary shifts, weight fluctuations, changes in physical activity, and significant life events like pregnancy or menopause can all influence the body's response to thyroid medication. Communicating these changes to healthcare providers is crucial, as they may necessitate adjustments in medication type or dosage. This continuous communication is key to ensuring that the treatment remains effective and responsive to the patient's changing needs.

A strong, collaborative relationship with healthcare providers is instrumental in the effective management of thyroid disorders. Open communication about symptom changes, lifestyle adjustments, and concerns about the treatment plan is essential. Patients should feel comfortable discussing different treatment options, including various types of thyroid medications, and understanding the advantages and limitations of each. This collaborative approach ensures that treatment decisions are well-informed and tailored to the individual's unique circumstances.

Treatment strategies for thyroid disorders should be highly personalized, taking into account factors like the type of thyroid disorder, age, weight, other health conditions, and personal treatment preferences. Regular follow-up appointments are crucial in this process, allowing for the assessment of the treatment's effectiveness and the opportunity for necessary adjustments. This ensures that the treatment remains aligned with the patient's evolving health status and provides the best possible outcome.

Empowering patients through education and self-advocacy is a vital aspect of managing thyroid health. Patients should be well-informed about their medications, including how to take them, potential side effects, and interactions with other substances. Encouraging patients to actively participate in their healthcare, ask questions, and seek second opinions when necessary, fosters a sense of control and involvement in their treatment journey. This empowerment is essential for successful long-term management of thyroid disorders.

Coping with Chronic Illness

Living with a chronic thyroid disorder encompasses not only physical health management but also navigating the emotional and psychological challenges that arise. The initial phase following diagnosis can be particularly tumultuous, as individuals grapple with a mix of emotions — relief at having an explanation for their symptoms juxtaposed with anxiety about managing a lifelong condition. This emotional rollercoaster often includes stages of grief and acceptance, as individuals come to terms with their new reality.

It's common to experience a spectrum of emotions, including frustration, sadness, and even anger, as one adjusts to the chronic nature of their condition. Thyroid disorders, due to their direct impact on metabolism, energy, and mood, contribute to ongoing emotional challenges. Fluctuations in thyroid hormone levels can lead to mood swings, periods of depression, or heightened anxiety, making emotional stability a challenging goal. This instability can have far-reaching effects on personal relationships and daily functioning.

Moreover, thyroid-related mood disorders, such as depression in hypothyroidism or anxiety in hyperthyroidism, add an additional layer of complexity to emotional well-being. Cognitive effects are also prevalent; issues with memory, focus, and concentration can be frustrating and affect various aspects of life, including work and personal relationships.

Developing a strong support system is crucial for those dealing with thyroid disorders. Support from family and friends provides not just emotional comfort but also a practical assistance network. Open communication about one's experiences and needs is key to nurturing these relationships. Additionally, connecting with others through thyroid disorder support groups, whether in-person or online, offers a unique form of empathy and understanding. Sharing experiences and coping strategies in these groups can provide comfort and practical advice, easing the sense of isolation that often accompanies chronic illness.

Professional support plays a vital role in managing the psychological impact of chronic thyroid conditions. Engaging with mental health professionals for therapy can offer effective coping mechanisms for stress, anxiety, and depression. Therapeutic approaches like cognitive-behavioral therapy can be particularly beneficial in dealing with the psychological challenges of living with a thyroid disorder. Patient advocacy groups and thyroid health organizations also serve as valuable resources, offering educational materials, support, and guidance. These groups often facilitate a deeper understanding of the condition and empower individuals to advocate for their health needs effectively.

Lifestyle adjustments and self-care are integral to coping with a thyroid disorder. Stress management techniques such as meditation, yoga, and mindfulness are beneficial for emotional regulation. Maintaining a healthy lifestyle, including a balanced diet, regular exercise, and sufficient sleep, is crucial for both physical and mental health.

Nutritional choices can directly influence thyroid function and overall well-being, while physical activity and sleep play significant roles in emotional health and stress management. Being informed and educated about one's condition is empowering. Understanding the nature of thyroid disorders, treatment options, and lifestyle factors that affect thyroid health can help reduce feelings of helplessness and encourage a proactive approach to health management.

In summary, coping with a chronic thyroid disorder requires a comprehensive approach that addresses the emotional and psychological challenges, builds a supportive network, and incorporates lifestyle adjustments and self-care practices. Through a combination of personal strategies, professional support, and community resources, individuals can effectively manage the complexities of their condition, maintaining a good quality of life and overall well-being.

Advocacy and Empowerment

Advocacy and empowerment in managing thyroid health are pivotal elements that go beyond mere treatment compliance. They involve a deep understanding of the condition, proactive engagement in healthcare decisions, and the effective use of resources and support systems. The journey begins with acquiring a thorough understanding of thyroid physiology and the specifics of various thyroid disorders. This knowledge base should encompass how the thyroid functions, the implications of hormonal imbalances, and the symptoms and signs of different thyroid conditions like hypothyroidism, hyperthyroidism, thyroiditis, and thyroid cancer.

It's crucial for patients to recognize how these conditions manifest in their bodies and understand the potential health implications. Staying informed about the latest research and developments in thyroid health is essential. Patients should actively seek up-to-date information from credible medical sources and participate in educational opportunities such as patient forums, health webinars, and conferences. This continuous learning process helps in understanding emerging treatment options and advancements in thyroid care.

Additionally, patients should be well-versed in the various treatment modalities available, including different types of thyroid hormone replacements, their dosing, side effects, and potential interactions with other medications or conditions. Knowledge of integrative approaches like diet modifications, supplements, and stress management techniques that complement traditional treatments is also beneficial.

Effective self-monitoring is a key aspect of empowerment. Patients should be adept at tracking their symptoms, understanding how to adjust lifestyle factors, and recognizing warning signs of thyroid imbalance. Keeping a symptom diary can be a helpful tool. Integrating lifestyle changes, such as a thyroid-supportive diet, regular exercise, and effective stress management strategies, is crucial in enhancing overall well-being and managing thyroid health.

Engaging with healthcare providers collaboratively and assertively is a critical component of advocacy. Effective communication skills are essential to convey concerns, symptoms, and preferences clearly. Patients should be prepared for medical appointments, and equipped with questions and discussion points. Building a trusting and respectful relationship with healthcare providers enables more personalized and effective care. In complex cases, seeking specialized care from endocrinologists or thyroid specialists can provide deeper insights and expertise.

Navigating the healthcare system efficiently is an integral part of advocacy. This involves understanding health insurance policies, patient rights, and how to access specialist care. Managing one's health records, including keeping track of medical appointments, test results, and medication histories, ensures preparedness and facilitates coordinated care among various healthcare providers.

Additionally, engaging with thyroid health communities and advocacy groups can provide access to a wealth of resources, including expert advice, patient experiences, and support networks. Peer support groups offer emotional backing, practical daily living tips, and a sense of belonging to a community of individuals who share similar experiences.

In conclusion, advocacy and empowerment in thyroid health management encompass a comprehensive approach that includes extensive education about the disorder, proactive engagement in healthcare decisions, effective communication with medical professionals, and leveraging community resources and support systems. By embracing these practices, individuals with thyroid disorders are better equipped to navigate their health journey, ensuring they receive optimal care and maintain a high quality of life.

Conclusion

As we bring this comprehensive exploration of thyroid health to a close, it's vital to reflect upon the journey we've embarked upon, rich with insights and lessons about managing and living with thyroid disorders. This book has been a voyage through the complexities of thyroid health, designed not just to inform but to empower you with a deeper understanding and a sense of control over your health journey.

Throughout the chapters, we've delved into the intricate details of thyroid disorders, exploring their physiological underpinnings, the subtleties of diagnosis, and the spectrum of symptoms that patients may experience. We've tackled the often-daunting world of treatments, from conventional medical approaches to the integrative therapies that can complement them. A significant focus has been on the criticality of regular monitoring and testing — an essential aspect that helps in fine-tuning treatment and ensuring effective management of the condition.

Adjusting to medication and treatment changes is a challenging yet crucial part of managing thyroid health. We've looked into how to recognize when adjustments are necessary and the importance of maintaining an open and collaborative relationship with healthcare providers. This process is not just about medical compliance but about understanding one's body, recognizing the nuances of changes in symptoms, and advocating for one's health needs.

Beyond the physical aspects, we've addressed the emotional and psychological terrain of living with a thyroid disorder. Coping with the chronic nature of thyroid conditions, the fluctuations in mood and energy, and the impact on one's mental well-being and self-image are aspects often overshadowed by physical symptoms. We discussed building strong support networks, engaging with communities, and seeking professional mental health support as essential strategies to navigate these challenges.

Empowerment through knowledge has been a recurring theme. Understanding your condition, being well-informed about treatment options, and making educated decisions about your health care are empowering acts. This empowerment is further amplified by actively participating in your health journey — asking questions, seeking clarifications, and being a part of the decision-making process in consultations with healthcare professionals.

Looking ahead, the landscape of thyroid health and treatment continues to evolve. Advances in medical research are continuously reshaping our understanding of thyroid disorders and opening new avenues for more effective treatments. Staying informed about these developments is crucial for anyone managing a thyroid condition. The future holds promise for improved management strategies, more personalized treatment approaches, and a deeper understanding of the interplay between thyroid function and overall health.

In closing, I offer words of encouragement and hope. Managing a thyroid disorder is a journey that requires resilience, adaptability, and persistence. While challenges are part and parcel of this journey, they are surmountable with the right tools, information, and support. Remember that you are an integral part of your healthcare team, and your active participation can significantly influence your treatment outcomes and quality of life. With each new day comes the opportunity for growth, learning, and moving closer to wellness.

May the knowledge and insights gained from this book serve as a guiding light, empowering you to navigate your thyroid health journey with confidence and optimism. Your path may have its twists and turns, but armed with knowledge, support, and a proactive attitude, you are well-equipped to face them. Keep moving forward with hope, knowing that each step you take is a step towards better health and well-being.